My RA Story

*Personal accounts of living with
rheumatoid arthritis*

My RA Story

*Personal accounts of living with
rheumatoid arthritis*

Edited by Brian Lynch
Introduction by Sinéad Moriarty

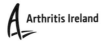
Arthritis Ireland

First published 2019 by Arthritis Ireland
1 Clanwilliam Square, Grand Canal Quay, Dublin 2 D02 DH77
www.arthritisireland.ie

ISBN 978-1-5272-4736-9

1 3 5 7 9 8 6 4 2

Cover design by Anú Design
Printed by Chameleon Print Management

This book is supported by a grant from MSD

Contents

Foreword

Welcome to *My RA Story*. This book is a collection of personal accounts of living with rheumatoid arthritis (RA). The purpose of this book is to increase awareness and understanding of RA, of what it is like to live with this chronic condition with its invisible pain and life-changing impact. It is also about giving hope to the thousands of people in Ireland who are living with this condition. Crucially, we also wish to provide a resource for people who are newly diagnosed with the disease and uncertain of what the future holds.

RA is an autoimmune disease in which the body's immune system – which normally protects its health by attacking foreign substances like bacteria and viruses – mistakenly attacks the joints. When this happens, the joints can become stiff and inflamed and cause pain. If this goes unchecked, the result is damage to the joints. That is why early intervention is vital.

Early diagnosis is key to better long-term outcomes. While symptoms of RA can vary from person to person, the most common are pain and swelling in the joints, stiffness in the joints, redness, inflammation and fatigue. RA can have a considerable impact on people's quality of life, particularly in relation to their career, relationships, lifestyle and mental health. These are the invisible effects of living with the disease.

Every year, over 2,000 people are diagnosed with RA in Ireland. In total, RA affects 45,000 people in this country; 70% of whom are women, three in four are of working age. For someone newly diagnosed with rheumatoid arthritis, coming to terms with the news can seem overwhelming. While there may be relief in being able to name what is wrong, there is also acknowledgement that RA is a chronic life-long condition, for which there is no cure. Such a dramatic shift in life circumstance can impact one's physical and mental well-being. It can be overwhelming trying to filter the volumes of information, assess what is trustworthy and relate to at a human level.

People have long feared RA as one of the most disabling types of arthritis. The good news is that the outlook has greatly improved for many people with newly diagnosed RA. Of course, RA remains a serious disease, and one that can vary widely in symptoms and outcomes. Even so, treatment advances have made it possible to stop or at least slow the progression of joint damage. Rheumatologists now have many new treatments that target the inflammation that RA causes. They also understand better when and how to use treatments to get the best results.

People's experiences of these treatments is a thread that runs through many of the stories in this collection. The reader will note that terms like DMARD (disease-modifying anti-rheumatic drug), NSAID (non-steroidal anti-inflammatory drug) and biologic crop up regularly. Anyone who wishes to get accessible, scientific and impartial information about these treatments is directed to websites and resources like those produced by Arthritis Ireland, the Health Products Regulatory Authority (HPRA) and the European Medicines Agency (EMA).

While medical advances have been made in the treatment of RA, we in Arthritis Ireland have been working relentlessly to support people living with arthritis and to improve their quality of life. In fact, that very phrase, 'people living with arthritis' underlines that arthritis is not just a disease that affects the person with the condition – the 'patient', if you like. Instead, there is a much wider circle also living with arthritis – family, work colleagues, team members – anyone who is impacted by this chronic condition. The ripple effect of the disease is much greater, therefore, than those experiencing the pain, fatigue, disruption and destruction of arthritis.

The funds raised through the sale of this book will help to further our work in providing services and information to people with RA here in Ireland.

I would like to thank everyone who took the time to write about their personal journey with RA. By sharing your story – the good, the bad and the ugly – you are helping to raise awareness of this often misunderstood disease and reduce the emotional isolation that many people diagnosed feel every day.

Gráinne O'Leary
Chief Executive

Introduction

Since being diagnosed with RA four years ago, I have found that talking to other people and writing about it has helped enormously.

It is only by talking to others with RA that I got through those first few dark and difficult years. It was by listening to other people's stories and experiences that I was able to figure out how to best manage the condition.

I feel very strongly that we need to raise awareness about this condition and get people to talk to each other and connect with others.

It can be a very lonely place and just being able to talk to someone who 'gets it' can be incredibly helpful and consoling and informative.

My journey with RA began in May 2015 when my dad dropped dead of a heart-attack on holidays in Spain. My siblings and I flew out to be with Mum and help organise getting the body flown home.

As I went to bed that first night in Spain, I noticed that my left knee had blown up. I thought it was air pressure on the plane or maybe I'd twisted it. I had a lot of other things on my mind, so I ignored it.

In the weeks and months after the funeral I began to feel really unwell. Terrible night sweats, no appetite and a tiredness that no amount of sleep could help. I was freezing all the time during the day and my eyes were constantly irritable. My knee continued to remain swollen.

I presumed I was getting the menopause. I went to my GP to get blood tests and planned to start HRT. Three days later the GP rang and said my blood tests were off the charts and she had made me an urgent appointment to see a rheumatologist.

I had never heard of a rheumatologist, but I duly went along. I still wasn't particularly worried, I've never been ill and have a fairly healthy lifestyle. I presumed he'd give me a pill and I'd be as good as new in no time.

He looked at my blood test result, and then at me and I was admitted to hospital then and there. I began to go downhill fast. After a week of non-stop poking prodding and over 40 blood tests, I was finally diagnosed with rheumatoid arthritis. I had no knowledge of what this meant so I googled it:

'RA is a chronic autoimmune disease that causes severe inflammation of the joints. There is no cure'

As I lay in hospital staring up at the ceiling on that long dark night, I remember thinking, 'This is what it feels like to be terrified.' I finally understood the true meaning of the word 'terror'.

Sleep evaded me as my mind tried to process what was happening. I didn't understand how a 'healthy' person could suddenly be so unwell.

As I lay in that dark hospital room I panicked. What did having RA mean? What was my future? Would I die? Would I be crippled for life? Would I be able to look after my kids? Would I have chronic pain for the rest of my life? Would this ruin my family's life?

I began to google and my fear grew worse. I went from never having had a panic attack in my life, to having them all the time. Big ones, long ones, frightening ones.

I seemed to have a very aggressive form of RA. Every consultant – and there were many – who came into my hospital room muttered 'Oh my goodness' and 'So aggressive!' when they looked at my chart.

The consultant said 'We need to fight fire with fire'; they gave me the highest doses of medicine and injections.

But despite all of the drugs, my left knee continued to flare-up. I then had 10 steroid injections into my knee (one a week). No difference. So, I was put on high doses of oral steroids. I remained on them for almost a year.

At one point my local pharmacist took me aside and asked me if I was sure that the high doses of meds I was on were correct. She looked extremely concerned. I nodded, unable to speak because I wanted to weep.

I spent hours in waiting rooms, having treatment, consultations, watching experts shaking their heads and using the words 'aggressive', 'unusual' and 'unfortunate' over and over again. I spent a lot of time weeping behind potted plants outside consultant rooms. I panicked, I paced up and down in the wee hours of the morning, I cried a lot and I worried *all* the time.

The loneliness is very challenging. No matter how wonderful your friends and family are – and mine really are – you are alone with your illness and your fears and concerns. At 3am it's just you and your thoughts. You and your mind conjuring awful outcomes. You and your pain. No one can possibly understand how you feel, you barely understand it yourself. You live inside your head as you try to process the shock and come to terms with a lifelong condition. It's a very lonely place.

But it was by going out and seeking advice from other people with RA that I began to really understand the condition and felt less alone. I met and spoke to the most wonderful people. Friends of friends, people's mothers in law, brothers in law, colleagues, cousins … anyone who had RA or knew anything about it.

I lost myself in those first few years after my diagnosis. I was nervous, frightened and overwhelmed. I hated not being able to go for a walk with my kids. I hated being utterly exhausted all the time. I felt old, miserable, crippled and useless.

I tried to do mindfulness courses and meditation but, in the end, I realised that it was only by talking to others and writing that I was able to come to terms with it all.

For a while, RA shattered my confidence in life and made me wary of the future. But I think it's vital that I learn something from this experience. I've accepted it and that has been a huge help. I've stopped asking how this happened and started asking what can I do to live the best life possible?

I take each day as it comes and am so very grateful for what I have. I know what a blessing health is and I will never take it for granted.

Let's keep talking to each other, encouraging each other and sharing information. By raising awareness and talking about RA, we can really help each other and our loved ones to understand this complex condition.

Sinéad Moriarty

Mary Banks

I don't think there's a 'one size fits all' way of living your life with RA, I can only tell how it has been for me. Many years ago, I watched a documentary about survivors of the Holocaust. Some survivors could only make sense of their lives by constantly talking about their experience and others could only make a life for themselves by never talking about their experience. Some of us are sharers, some of us ain't. Being of the non-sharing variety, for me to talk about bad stuff is to make it into something much bigger. I don't want to make bad stuff any bigger than it needs to be. The bad stuff is over, so I can talk about it now.

Stuff of history

My RA was a creeper. I am now 60 and the flare-ups began in my early twenties before I had a car. My memory of pain begins at a bus stop and my wonder at why and how the gusting wind was causing my ankle so much grief. My left ankle continued swelling up, on and off, every few months and I thought I must have twisted it one time in the melee of getting on the bus to work.

I also remember heading into town on Saturday mornings and having to head for the bus home after 15 minutes of walking because my feet hurt. The silly thing is, around this

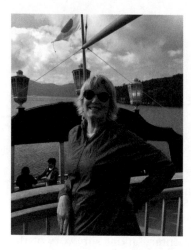

Mary Banks

time, my eldest brother had been diagnosed with psoriatic arthritis and my uncle had RA, but it never entered my head that this might be something similar. I didn't mention it to anybody.

Fast forward to age 30, I came down with what I thought was the flu, but a month later, still had muscle ache and painful joints. I was now definitely suspicious that it might be RA and went to a doctor near my workplace (I didn't have a GP). He told me it was probably still the flu and to keep taking painkillers.

A month later, I went back to him as the pain was worse; I had greater difficulty walking, using my hands, extending my arms. I told him of my suspicion and about my brother and uncle. I asked for a blood test for rheumatoid factor. He explained to me the statistics of rheumatoid factor and how it didn't make for a definitive diagnosis and finished by saying, 'You don't really want a blood test do you?'

Every fact he told me was correct, but I felt devastated by his last words and I regret that I didn't have the gumption to say 'Yes, I do want that test!' I left his surgery thinking I was a tense, anxious hypochondriac.

I can't blame him for my way of thinking or my nature, but I still wonder why he said that. He was a very young doctor, so I have, kind of, forgiven him. I'd forgive him more if I could forget!

For the next four years I put up with the flare-ups, oscillating between the thought that I was a tense individual and therefore inflicting this pain and stiffness on myself and the other thought that 'no' this was definitely RA. I couldn't bring myself to go to another GP and be told the same thing – that RA was unlikely – because that would mean it really was my fault. I am ashamed of how lacking in courage I was at that time.

Now 34 and at a workplace medical screening for staff, I plucked up the courage to tell a nurse my story. She was very direct and told me that the medical profession is no different to any other profession; some people are good at their job and others aren't. She said I had the signs and all the symptoms of RA, as well as a family history and to get myself to another GP immediately.

I found a lovely GP and she immediately referred me to St Vincent's rheumatology unit and I was definitively diagnosed. An immense relief.

Bad stuff
Pain One: a heavy aching muscle and joint pain and stiffness all over. My body is leaden.

Pain Two: the pain of inflammation, skin swollen and red hot and sensitive like sunburned skin.

Pain Three: a severe, gasp-out-loud pain, as if all the bones in my body are broken and the most insignificant of movements such as flicking my fringe out of my eyes causes some of those bones to grate.

All these pains exist in unison.

Typical bad old day: Alarm goes off three hours before I need to head out front door. Struggle to reach painkillers and lift glass of water. Swallow. Slump back and wait an hour. Pain eased a little, roll to edge of bed and try to sit up without putting pressure on hands, wrists or elbows. Manoeuvre legs over edge and put feet on floor.

Now picture the Pink Panther, crouched forward and saying 'Ouch, ouch …. ouch, ouch' as he gingerly propels one foot in front of the other towards the shower. The bliss of an electric shower – the hot water doesn't run out. I would stand there until I felt everything loosen a little and when I was more upright and a now pinker Pink Panther I'd exit.

I learned to leave the lid off all toiletries and to walk downstairs sideways and to leave all internal doors open so I could access rooms in the morning. The next time you butter a slice of toast have a look at how your fingers, hand and wrist operate; such a variety of movement. After a struggle I could get butter on the knife, but not from there onto the toast, too much variety of movement for those broken bones.

Some days it was easier to walk to work than drive the car, depressing the clutch or changing gear were just not possible. But that long, slow walk would loosen up my body even more, so then I could get on with my day. The trick was to keep moving. When I'd get home in the evening I would seize up again.

Fever. I learned to double-up on mattress covers after the Shroud of Turin incident when, after a bout of fever, I removed the single cover to discover my upper body outline in a beautiful sepia tone on the mattress.

Fatigue. This was hard because if I succumbed and rested I then had to go through the 'get myself going' routine above.

The embarrassment of it all. It's okay to be creaky at 60, but I found it mortifying at 30.

Drug stuff

Today science and the study of biomarkers means that aggressive treatment can begin immediately with the effect that the disease can be brought under control quickly with minimal chance of joint damage. In the early '90s it was different. A softly, softly approach with a build up over the years to the hard stuff, if the RA kept progressing.

I started out on an anti-inflammatory (NSAID) for a number of years. It helped reduce inflammation and pain and I still use it at times when I know I'll be doing a lot of standing, but the RA continued its progression and following a particularly bad flare-up I was put on a different NSAID for six months and then a DMARD (disease-modifying anti-rheumatic drug). Life was definitely more manageable on the DMARD, but I hated it, as it made me nauseous for two days every week. I switched to taking it by injection, but same story.

The funny thing is the same drug doesn't knock a feather out of my brother, even though we're from the same gene pool. I think biomarkers must be like fingerprints, unique to each individual.

And so it continued for about 15 years, ups and downs, not quite under control but manageable. Then about six years ago, the RA went rogue.

Luckily for me it was around the time of a scheduled appointment at Vincent's because I don't know that I wouldn't again have dithered about calling attention to it. I was prescribed an anti-TNF therapy. I could call this biologic drug 'miraculous' except for the fact that it isn't, it is the result of wonderful science.

Within two weeks of taking this drug, all of my symptoms began to disappear and my knuckles began to reappear.

For a few years I injected the DMARD weekly and injected the biologic fortnightly. I no longer take the DMARD, which means I'm free of weekly nausea, but I am grateful for the years it got me by. I have anti-inflammatories and painkillers on standby for the 'on the razz' days. I continue to inject the biologic fortnightly. I HAVE NOT HAD A FLARE-UP SINCE!

Good stuff

The silver lining to doing my best to ignore bad stuff is that I unknowingly trained my brain to keep the pain walking three paces behind me. I knew I had this cracked when, two hours into a long car drive, I noticed my right hand was resting in my lap. Only then did I become conscious of the pain in my hand. My brain had subconsciously registered the pain and removed my hand from the steering wheel to help ease it.

A diagnosis of RA does not mean a life of doom and gloom. I now go to exercise classes twice a week (my heart hoorays if the class is cancelled), I regularly walk 5k and I travel to the ends of the earth with my lovely biologic drug in my very cool coolbag designed to keep it at the correct temperature. When your RA is under control or even semi under control, life can be manageable, good and even great if you are proactive in getting the pain to walk three paces behind you.

Stuff I've learned

That stoicism can be taken too far. It is better to complain, to say 'ouch!' out loud. Be honest about pain levels and 'fess up when things get too much for you. GPs and consultants aren't psychic.

In hindsight I've learned that all of my big flare-ups

started a few months after a difficult time. Some stressors are outside our control, the tribulations of life. It is important to pay attention to your health at these times, to anticipate a flare-up. Other stressors are things that are within our control. We do so many things that are stressful to us because we feel duty bound to or because we don't want to let others down. It is better for your health to say 'no'. It gets easier with practice.

That prophylactic doesn't always mean condom. For me it means swallowing anti-inflammatories and painkillers in anticipation of the pain I expect to get because I'm going to be on my feet all day. I no longer wait for the pain to begin.

Stuff I'm grateful for

I'm grateful that I did not have a more severe form of RA.

I'm grateful that the menopause completely passed me by because I attributed any symptoms to RA.

In the bad old days, I'd console myself by thinking 'I'm grateful that I'm not an orchestra conductor/jogger/surgeon/tennis player, etc. because then this would be so much worse'.

I'm grateful my passion is reading – it involves very little movement.

I'm grateful for the invention of e-readers because they are easier to hold than a book.

I'm grateful that I'm alive in the time of 'athleisure wear'. Thick soled ugly shoes are now edgy!

I'm extremely grateful that my biologic is paid for under the Drugs Payment Scheme.

Most of all I'm grateful to everybody at St Vincent's Hospital rheumatology unit; I'd be a very sad human being without their care.

Tom Barrett

My story starts in September 1980, just three weeks after my twenty-first birthday, when I started to develop slight pains in my left shoulder. I wasn't overly concerned as I had just started back weight training for athletics and I put the pain down to just overdoing it at the previous training session. At the time I was extremely fit, as I had just completed a reasonably successful athletics season competing in the short sprints and long and triple jumps. I had been competing in athletics since I was 11 years of age.

It was after a few days, when the pain had gotten worse instead of improving and I started to lose the function in the shoulder, that I decided to go to the family doctor. I hadn't seen a GP for years; this doctor was elderly and, thinking back, probably did not have a lot of knowledge of rheumatoid arthritis.

After an injection into the shoulder I was as good as ever after a few days, so I continued with my weight training. After about six weeks the symptoms returned, so off to the GP who repeated the process. Recovery took place similar to the first time. This time, symptoms returned after five weeks; back to the GP who repeated the process.

Maybe there was poor communication between the GP and myself, as I had continued training once the pain had

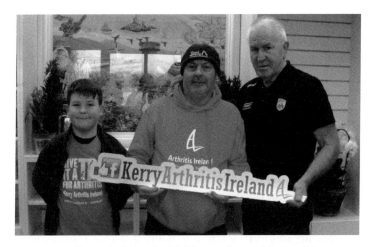

Tom Barrett (centre) pictured with his grandson, Jaidon, and former government minister and Kerry football legend, Jimmy Deenihan

subsided. When the pain came back, it had started to spread to other parts of my body and at this stage I definitely was not able to train. As I had just gotten my first job after finishing college, I wanted to hold on to it and in the end I was getting an injection every second night just to keep me going. Unfortunately, I was unable to continue working and had to give up the job.

A few months earlier, my whole focus was on what I needed to do to have a chance of breaking the long-standing Irish long jump record. This focus changed drastically when I lost a lot of weight, was in extreme pain all over my body and barely able to walk. I was just about able to lift a cup of tea to my mouth and that was using both hands. I could feel and see that whatever illness I had was wreaking havoc on my body.

My main concern was will I survive and if so will I still be able to walk.

It was roughly six months later that a cardiologist at Kerry General Hospital diagnosed RA. I say cardiologist because consultant rheumatologists were pretty scarce on the ground at this time. Not alone did I not know what RA entailed, but it was very difficult to get any relevant information on the condition, never mind having the option of getting practical support, the kind which Arthritis Ireland and its local branches provide nowadays.

At the time, I got a pamphlet on RA from the local branch of The Arthritis Foundation of Ireland, the forerunner to Arthritis Ireland. Even though this was the best information that was available at the time, it only caused me to have more questions, to which I could find no answers at the time.

Eventually, after starting anti-inflammatory medication, getting some steroid injections and visiting a rheumatologist in Cork and a second one in Dublin, I gradually started to regain control of my body. I returned to work about 12 months later, despite having lost a lot of function in most of my joints and I was still in a lot of pain.

In the following 10 years, I functioned reasonably well. I kept annoying my GP to keep trying new medications; I kept active; used wrist supports, sometimes a crutch, joint strapping, physiotherapy – anything I thought that would give me an edge over my arch enemy RA.

I have now learned that this is a very vulnerable time in the life of a person living with chronic arthritis as unscrupulous manufacturers of products that claim to cure arthritis take advantage of the vulnerability of people who would do anything to get rid of their unrelenting pain and stiffness.

Also during this period, I got married, became the father of two boys and a girl, and achieved a BA in Public Management. My wife Deborah was a great support as she took responsibility for the kids, home, as well as taking care of me during bad flare-ups and hospital stays. Having this extra support can be the deciding factor between gaining control of your arthritis and just barely coping.

The biggest change in my RA came a few years later when I changed rheumatologists and was put on a combination of painkillers and anti-inflammatories, as well as DMARDs (disease-modifying anti-rheumatic drugs) and biologics, rather than just anti-inflammatories on their own.

It was also around the same time that I got involved in setting up the Kerry branch of Arthritis Ireland, which was comprised of local volunteers, all of whom were living with arthritis. I trained as a Living Well with Arthritis course leader, with the main aim of giving support to people like myself who are looking for relevant information on how to manage their condition.

It was only then that I discovered the true severity of RA. I was well aware that due to the pain of inflamed joints and surrounding tissues, people with arthritis are unable to function normally in their everyday lives; living a life with limited mobility can be very frustrating and depressing.

The inflammatory process that underlies inflammatory type arthritis not only affects the joints, but other parts of the body as well. Pain, swelling, fatigue, malaise, fever, cognitive dysfunction, memory issues, weight loss and depression are common non-joint symptoms or side effects of having rheumatoid arthritis.

We also have comorbidities to deal with, which exacerbate our symptoms. Lung, heart and kidney disease are all more prevalent in people with inflammatory arthritis compared with the general population. Pain isn't always the most persistent or bothersome symptom either — it can be fatigue. Every case of arthritis is different for the person living with it.

Discovering these facts helped me understand the reasons why I had developed secondary issues with my eyes, lungs and heart, as well as other complications as a direct consequence of my RA. Many years of taking exceptionally strong medications had also had an impact.

What do these complications look like? Well, after three total hip replacements on my left hip – the first when I was 31 – leaving me with a very pronounced limp, two wrist fusions, emergency surgery for a perforated duodenal ulcer which gave rise to a second surgery for a very large abdominal hernia which has left me with a permanent pot belly-like stomach, secondary Sjögren's syndrome, osteopenia and mitral valve prolapse. This is only my top seven; if I listed everything you would be reading forever!

I believe that people living with chronic arthritis have a close relationship and affiliation with Christ and some of the saints in that we all understand the meaning of pain and suffering.

Inflammatory arthritis is like an iceberg, in that only one-third is visible to the ordinary eye and the other two-thirds which cause the greatest amount of the damage are unseen. Not only does RA assault your physical wellbeing, but it also infringes on your mental state of mind. In my own case, I look the picture of health, just like many others living with RA; but the expression 'never judge a book by its cover' could not be more accurate.

Research proves that doing appropriate exercise on a regular basis helps with the management of arthritis, rather than causing more damage to your joints. I trained as a walking leader and set up a branch walking group in Tralee. Shortly afterwards, also on behalf of the Kerry branch of Arthritis Ireland, I set up hydrotherapy classes run by a chartered physiotherapist. The benefits gained by the participants were amazing, so much so that demand for aqua classes resulted in us switching from hydrotherapy classes to running aqua aerobics and aqua jogging classes in the local sports centre. Since then the branch has added 'Step 2 the Beat' dance and 'Gym-Theraband' strengthening exercise classes to their exercise programmes list.

I believe that becoming a volunteer with the local branch of Arthritis Ireland gave me the opportunity to organise events which benefited me as much as it benefited others living with arthritis. Had I taken the easy option and waited for others to organise these events, I might still be waiting!

There is something about volunteering that makes you feel good, as well as giving you something else to think about rather than your own arthritis. Volunteering is also an excellent way of getting to know and becoming known to health care professionals.

If like me, you want to take back control of your arthritis then you need to be prepared to endure a period of trial and error to find the right medication, or mix of medications, that works best for you. Even when I found the right mix, managing my condition was still a daily struggle as the unpredictability of the condition caused me to have good and bad days, so I still have to continue working hard at maintaining a healthy lifestyle to minimize how RA affects me daily.

Proper management of my RA did not come cheap. Taking back control was not easy and involved having to make tough choices and many family sacrifices: new treatments or that sun holiday or a new car. Being able to hold down a full-time job helped, as I was able to afford faster access to the many healthcare professionals, specialists and treatments which are so necessary if you want to regain total control of your arthritis. Unfortunately, not everybody will be in a similar position.

Remember that making the decision to do something about taking back control of your arthritis is solely your choice and nobody else's, and I mean nobody else can make that decision for you. It will not be easy to take that first step; but trust me it will be well worth the effort.

Mary Blake

My RA story began in the autumn of 2011. I had just returned from a cruise on the Mediterranean. I noticed I was getting quite stiff, especially when sitting down and attempting to get up from a chair. At first, I put it down to all the stairs I had climbed while on the cruise ship, but as time went on and I became less agile, I visited my GP.

He sent me for blood tests and the results showed that I had an inflammatory condition and he recommended I see a consultant. This came as a shock to me. I made an appointment to see a consultant rheumatologist. When I eventually got an appointment, the consultant told me that I did not have rheumatoid arthritis. He wrote to the GP recommending a drug I could take if I got worse.

My symptoms did in fact get worse and during the summer of 2012, I was in a lot of pain. I went to see a different consultant in September who told me quite categorically that I did indeed have RA and I would have to take an immune system suppressant. As I have quite a sensitive stomach, she agreed to let me do this by injection. I had to have a number of x-rays before beginning the drug, so could not start the treatment straight away. While I was waiting to begin treatment, I signed up to do the Living Well with Arthritis course. I found this very helpful, especially as I felt I was

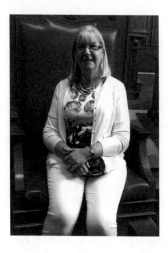

Mary Blake

embarking on the unknown. Some of the participants who were ahead of me on their treatment path assured me that once on the drug my symptoms would improve. I felt very reassured by this.

I began the treatment in January 2013. I have to inject myself once a week, which is not pleasant. However, my symptoms did improve over time and thankfully I have been able to reduce the dosage. I am also lucky that this DMARD (disease-modifying anti-rheumatic drug) works for me and I have not required a second immunosuppressant.

I find living with RA manageable, but quite difficult at times. I was not able to work for the last seven years, as I am unable to sit or stand for any length of time. In the beginning, the side effects of the medication were quite debilitating, causing nausea, headaches and fatigue. I was on an invalidity pension and you are not allowed to work while on this. Apart from the loss of earnings, I find trying to fill-in time is very difficult.

I had always worked and had gone back to college and retrained and I feel I missed out on opportunities to put that training to good use. I am no longer on the invalidity pension, but I find my age is against me now in the search for employment, as is the length of time I have spent out of the workforce.

Apart from the physical side effects, another aspect of the medication which I find stressful is the necessity for three-monthly blood tests. I do not like hospitals and I feel having RA has plunged me into the world of hospitals and doctors.

Living with RA can affect other aspects of life which may not be so obvious. I can no longer wear high heels and if I am dressing for an occasion, I feel my outfit is incomplete as I do not feel 'dressed' in flats.

My balance is not as good as it was and I always have to hold on to rails when going down stairs. This can make one feel feeble. Also thinning hair can cause anxiety and embarrassment. Having to ask for help with chores can be frustrating and lots of packaging while purporting to be 'child proof' are in fact impossible for people with arthritis to open. Also travelling on public transport can at times be quite daunting, especially buses. By all appearances, I do not have anything wrong with me and it can be embarrassing if I am not able to stand for a journey or need to hold on to bars or wait for the bus to stop before getting up from the seat.

This is my story of living with RA to date. All in all, it is not easy, but it is manageable at the moment. Organisations such as Arthritis Ireland are very useful and sharing with and getting support from other people with the condition is very helpful. I hope and pray that a cure is found some day and, in the meantime, that my condition remains stable.

Peter Boyd

In the middle of delivering a very informative, and might I add entertaining, talk on arthritis, Arthritis Ireland and my journey with this life-changing condition, an elderly gent interrupted me with the best heckle, question and enquiry I've ever encountered.

'Son, why don't I like bananas?'

Stopped dead in my tracks explaining the difference between osteoarthritis and inflammatory forms of arthritis such as rheumatoid arthritis, I answered the only way I could: 'I don't know.'

Such a wonderfully simple and straight forward answer. I laughed as I spoke, not in a cruel mocking way, just together with a man who was genuinely puzzled as to why I didn't know the answer to his question.

Eight years ago, I sat with the same puzzled expression in front of doctor after doctor, in altogether more serious situations. Professional after professional told me they didn't know what was wrong with me or how it would impact on my future.

I worked as a barman in 2011. I had a bought a new home in 2008, had a new car and I had just started going out with a new girlfriend. I played 5-a-side football and golf, had plenty of disposable cash after paying the mortgage and

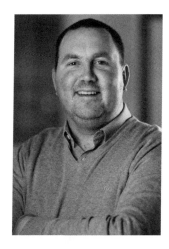

Peter Boyd

was blissfully ignorant of any struggles that might enter my 27-year-old life.

Early in 2011, I began to feel tired more often and struggled to recover between shifts. Working until late at night, followed by long day shifts and training hard in between, my body never recovered.

Presuming I was burning the candle at both ends, I didn't pay much heed to the fatigue. When the pain became unbearable, ignorance was no longer an option.

I couldn't lift crates of beer, I couldn't stand for hours on end, and I dreaded anyone ordering a bottle of cider off the bottom shelf of the fridge. My knees, hips and hands were in agony all day, every day and with no chance of recovery through sleep, the pain and fatigue multiplied.

It all came to a head on a Saturday evening in June 2011, when after a busy day I was chatting to a couple at the counter. I was in so much pain and so drained of any energy, I fell asleep on the taps in front of me, mid-conversation, mid-shift.

My bosses saw me, I was incredibly embarrassed and

scared for my future career. They were fantastic though and offered me two weeks holidays, starting immediately, to rest, recuperate and recover before continuing my employment.

I never returned.

I was eventually diagnosed with rheumatoid arthritis and fibromyalgia after touring the specialists and departments of Dublin's hospitals. For two years the only thing I gained were new diagnoses (the final count was 11 separate conditions), while on the debit side, I was losing everything.

I pushed my girlfriend away first. I wasn't going to ask anyone to be my carer when the replacements and the surgeries started. There was no discussion, I simply decided that was the best path for both of us.

I've lost touch with some of the best friends in the world. When you're so tired and sore that you cancel plans late in the day too often, with the greatest will in the world, patience runs out and the invites dry up. It's only natural.

With no job, the money disappeared and so did my specially picked out car. I had no disposable income as I had to rely on handouts and benefits. I hated this, I had always worked and earned my money, I felt guilty taking benefits that were deservedly there to support me.

With each layer of materialism that was stripped away, my confidence and self-worth disappeared too. I was a burden on society, I was useless and on a personal level all I had to look forward to was pain, immobility, surgeries and replacements.

Everything got on top of me and became too much. Anxiety and depression built up; my future looked bleak to say the least.

Everybody told me that though rheumatoid arthritis was bad, it wouldn't kill me. All the symptoms are awful, but not enough to finish you off. I feel RA nearly killed me.

My anxiety and depression became so deep that I attempted suicide three times as a direct result of my diagnosis. Thankfully, with my low self-confidence and self-worth, I wasn't very good at that either.

I don't say this flippantly. Suicide is not something to joke about and I know how close I was to ending it all. It's important to see the depths of despair that RA can push a person to and realise the level of support needed on diagnosis.

Arthritis Ireland have been key to my rehabilitation and recovery.

My first contact was through a six-week self-management course where I realised there were other young people like me in the same position. When I followed that by volunteering on the helpline, I began to grow and mature further.

Realising that no matter how I felt I could provide support, information and a listening ear to those who felt vulnerable and lost was massive. Through the helpline, I rebuilt my confidence and self-worth; my disability allowance became 'pay' for my shifts on the phones.

Suddenly a new future opened in front of me.

I volunteered for everything in Arthritis Ireland, from the family fun days to sitting on the board of directors. Nobody should ever feel as lost and bereft as I did the day I got my diagnosis.

With a little confidence returning and faith that medication control was allowing me to be reliable on the helpline, I looked at other paths for the future.

A former fitness instructor and barman, I needed to do something completely different for the 30-odd years of work I had in front of me. Therefore, I returned to college in Dún Laoghaire and the feeling of being successful at something again was amazing.

Two years later, I emerged with two separate qualifications and two Student of the Year awards. I was doing something I enjoyed, I was doing something I was good at and with control over my RA, I was ready to take on the world again.

I continue to volunteer with Arthritis Ireland. I now deliver those same self-management courses, and little gives me as much pleasure as helping those who are in the same position as I was in 2011. I chair the research sub-committee of the board and I love being at the forefront of research that will one day ensure nobody goes down the path I did.

Another aspect of my volunteerism is Arthritis Ambassador talks. These involve meeting school and university groups, retirement groups, Men's Sheds, health professionals, anyone in fact, and discussing what arthritis is, how it affects tots to centenarians, and how we can learn to self-manage in conjunction with rheumatologists and doctors.

This is how I ended up in front of a nursing home crowd at the end of their health week being asked why someone else doesn't like bananas!

Thinking back on the journey I've taken since 2011, one could only laugh at the question and move on.

I've rebuilt my life from the ruins of that night eight years ago when I left the pub as an employee for the last time. I've overcome loss, survived and grown.

At this point in my life, I can say that despite the pain I continue to experience and everything I've gone through because of it, I'm grateful for rheumatoid arthritis.

I'm a more empathetic and understanding person than I was before. I realise there are hundreds of invisible illnesses that the person beside you on the train is silently braving out.

It's also given me the opportunity to speak to the media about an issue that affects one in four, had me fly to Brussels,

Zurich, Amsterdam and more to make speeches and present workshops, and led me to a new job and career I wouldn't have found, but which I love even more than I did bar-work.

Finally, it's made me the man I am today. The good, the bad and in between have been moulded by my RA and the journey I've been on.

The good must out-weigh the bad because I'm in love with the most beautiful woman in the world and, what's more, she loves me. All of me.

Arthritis, pain, fatigue, possible replacements in the future. She loves me and whatever happens we'll cope with it together.

Now how to explain to 2010 Peter an old man will ask me in 2019 why he doesn't like bananas...

Dee Brennan

It all started when I began waking up in the mornings and my knees were locked in a 90 degree angle, unable to straighten out. I would drag myself into my mom and dad's room by my arms, as my legs were too sore and stiff to walk. I was four years old.

I can only imagine how my parents felt seeing their young daughter unable to walk into their room in the morning and getting progressively worse. My mom used to run a hot bath for me on the mornings when it was really bad, and lay me in the bath to try allow the heat to work its magic and help to relieve the stiffness. From there, it was hospital appointment after hospital appointment with my mom by my side for every single one, trying to figure out what was causing my pain and swelling.

Eventually I was diagnosed with juvenile rheumatoid arthritis. I didn't understand at that age what it was or what impact it would have on my life.

After my first operation to remove fluid from my knee, I returned to school; I must have been in senior infants. I had a cast on my knee which the whole class signed. I remember the other children in my class saying that I had broken my leg, seeing that I was in a cast, and I believed that's what had happened to me, that I broke my leg. Even though no event

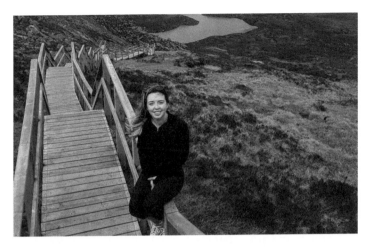

Dee Brennan

had caused it to be broken, it was just easier to comprehend at that age. I had a second operation at around age six, again to have fluid removed from the same knee.

My primary school in Cork was really understanding of my condition. On the cold winter mornings, I was allowed to bring my 'heat bunny' into school to warm in the microwave to put on my knees. In second class, I made it to Páirc Uí Chaoimh finals for running and that's when I thought my legs had gotten better. I was also involved in soccer and camogie with the local clubs growing up and until my teenage years, which I loved. However, sometimes my friends and I would go more for the chats than to play.

As confusing a time as secondary school is, having arthritis definitely made it more so. I didn't tell many new friends about it, as I thought it was too hard to explain and it's supposed to be 'an old person's disease'. However, close friends I would tell, as yearly flare-ups around the wintertime were a thing. I continued with my check-ups in Cork University Hospital around every three months and I was taking different medications. These included a DMARD (disease-modifying anti-rheumatic drug), anti-inflammatories and sometimes steroids.

To this day, when I think about that DMARD I get a bad taste in my mouth. The amount of the tablets I took fluctuated with how good or bad my joints were. I'm sure my parents and brother and sister could still tell you the weekly ordeal of sitting me down to take them. I absolutely hated them, they were very harsh on my tummy and I would feel nauseous for about a day or two afterwards.

I would be jealous of my brother and sister not having to take tablets and also wondered why I was the unlucky one?

I tried everything from putting the tablets into a spoonful of ice-cream to putting them into a chocolate muffin. Anything to mask the horribly toxic, chemical taste.

It wasn't until years later, when I jetted off on my J1, that my mom found a large stash of tablets in the lining of a cushion in my room. Ones that I had told my parents I had taken and then hid, or sometimes I would put them down the sink or toilet (sorry mom and dad). I would have preferred to be in pain rather than take them.

I gave up most team sports when I was in about fifth year, partially because I thought I wasn't good enough at them and partially because going into a clash with another hurley was extremely sore.

Doing my leaving cert was definitely a very stressful time, as everyone knows. But this stress was also heightened by me experimenting with different medications. I finally found my voice and told my parents and doctors that I would not continue to take the DMARD as I found it too toxic on my body. I tried taking that drug using syringes, however, that was even more of a horrific experience, so I stopped after a couple of weeks.

And then came the biologics. Learning how to inject yourself with medication is a very odd experience, and still to this day, just as I'm about to push the button of the injection, a little bit of fear kicks in, kind of like ripping off a plaster.

The first biologic I began around the time of the leaving cert and it had an immediate positive impact on my arthritis. Within weeks I felt the best I had ever felt! I remember going on my sixth year holiday with friends and sprinting up and down the beaches and doing various activities, and my friends saying how they hadn't seen me feeling so well in so long.

I began college in University College Cork in 2012 and also started my first ever part-time job that Christmas. Just when I thought things were looking up, is when they took a turn for the worst. My biologic injections started to lose their impact and the job I had which involved being on my feet all day was beginning to take its toll. I know people might wonder why I got a job where I had to stand all day when I knew it would cause me pain, but to be honest, I really wanted to be like all my other friends who had started making their own bit of money.

I remember one day leaving that job in floods of tears because of how much pain I was in. A one-minute walk to the bus stop was taking me more than five minutes, because I was taking each step so slowly and carefully and each step was more painful than the last. Climbing up and down the steps of the bus was excruciating and I kept my head buried in my hood so as not be seen by anyone.

I didn't want anyone to see the pain in my face and wonder why a 'normal' looking 18 year old was crying while walking onto the bus. My dad collected me that day and I still remember the look on his face when he saw the pain I was in. As if he would have done anything to take it away.

I made the decision that January to drop-out of college. It was taking too much out of me, physically and mentally.

The next couple of months are a bit of a blur. It was probably the worst flare-up I had experienced. It affected my sleep, as I would wake up to move positions and it could take my body a couple of minutes to cooperate with me wanting to move, as every joint had ceased up.

My mom has been my rock, for my entire life. With me for every appointment, every new medication, every blood test (I sat on her lap for blood tests until I was 12), and every up and down. I particularly remember around the time of this flare-up, the mornings being the worst. My mom would come down to my room and dress me. I couldn't reach down to put on my socks and knickers, as my knees wouldn't bend and I couldn't reach. My elbows, wrists and fingers were all inflamed.

We would joke about me being like an 80-year-old woman trapped in a 19 year old's body (with no disrespect, as there are probably 80 year olds who were more physically able than I was). Being able to make a light-hearted jokes made it all a bit easier.

My consultant in CUH then recommended I try a different biologic. I am now 25 years old, I have been on weekly injections of that drug for six years and I have not had a severe flare-up since. I finally found the medication that works for me.

I went back to college and graduated in 2017 with a BSc in Public Health and now work in an office job doing research. Don't get me wrong, I still experience pain in different ways most days. For example, even typing up my story, my wrists are beginning to become 'niggly' as I like to call it. I have trouble opening jars, kneeling and lifting. I become fatigued quite easily. My ankles hurt if I walk around for too long in unsupportive shoes. My lower back hurts if I stand for too long. My ankles and wrists become sore when I drive for long periods. My neck hurts if I don't sleep under two pillows. My whole body aches if I miss my injection by a day.

However, I'm also the healthiest I have ever been. I'm at the age where I want to take advantage of what my body *can do* instead of what it can't. I absolutely love keeping active and I try mostly to fuel my body with healthy foods. I love going to the gym, doing yoga, going for walks or hikes with friends, swimming, and stretching. And I know my body and my mind thank me for it.

For anyone who has been newly diagnosed with rheumatoid arthritis, I know how hard it can be. I would recommend being very open and honest with your peers or colleagues about the impact it has on you. There are so many supports out there in colleges and workplaces, you just need to ask. I also realise how tough flare-ups can be, and sometimes when going through it, exercising is the last thing you want to do and you think it will add to your pain. However, I've learned that not keeping physically active and not allowing your joints that movement can sometimes be even worse. Something like swimming can be hugely beneficial, as it takes the pressure off your joints, while also allowing you to be active.

Arthritis is unusual because you can't see it. And I have become very open to talking about it over the last few years and many people I have told have said things like 'I would never have thought you have arthritis' or 'You don't look like you have arthritis'. And they would be right. I don't look like I have arthritis, but it's something I live with and manage every day having tried different methods for years. It can be easier said than done, but I will continue to try my best to keep on top of it and hopefully help others along the way.

James Brosnan

My journey with RA started in 2008. I had a severe flu that just would not clear up and a chest pain with severe fatigue which finally ended up in a hospital stay. Despite many tests, there were no answers and after four days, I was discharged, told to rest and take paracetamol.

For the next two years and after meeting with many different consultants with hefty fees and various egos, I was told I had chronic fatigue syndrome, fibromyalgia, ME and the real beauty of 'It's all in your head' after my first visit to the 'top consultant in Ireland' (my GP's description). Take vitamin D and multivitamins was the recommendation after my second.

During the next two years I started running, ran marathons and was in great shape, bar a few niggles; but something still wasn't quite right.

Then in 2012, another knockout; this time severe fatigue and joint pain and I ended up back in hospital. More tests, more mystery, no answers. However, I was told that three years earlier on my last stay that I'd had pleurisy.

This finished me with the medical route and my faith in doctors. I was placed on medication to deal with fibromyalgia, but this did not sit well with me. Over the next 12 months, I weaned myself off them.

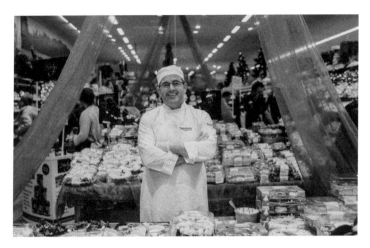

James Brosnan

I took care into my own hands; ate clean, cut out wheat, gluten, and dairy especially; took loads of different vitamins, tried lots of different alternative therapies with various results, even trained in one which gave me a perspective of what energy therapies do.

My symptoms abated and things improved, but the painful fatigue didn't really. Running a few miles felt like I'd run a marathon. That was a big loss to me and still is.

Then in the autumn of 2017, BANG, oh my God, the pains, the fatigue. Every joint ached, simple functions were a real effort. I continued to work as a baker, as the heat of the bakery was great to warm the muscles and joints, but everything else stopped.

My daily walk was stopped by the pains.

I continued until early January when I finally went to my GP and was put on steroids. I was referred to my local Bon Secours hospital in Tralee to a rheumatologist and within 20 minutes of my story I was diagnosed with RA. I asked how she knew, as this had not shown in previous tests. It turns out I'm seronegative, so it would never show in the many blood tests over the years. I started a treatment programme on DMARDs and finally started to see results over the next six to 12 months. Dr Buckley has been fantastic.

As part of my therapy, I started back in the gym which helped enormously, even though it was very tough at the start. I'm now very fit again, my joints have improved, my medications reduced, and I am able to walk a couple of miles. But I'm also listening to my body and doing as it tells me by not overdoing things. Work has reduced to a four-day week, with two days on at a time which has helped a lot. I really didn't think I'd be able to continue working after my last flare-up.

Life is good, symptoms are receding and hopefully will continue to do so; God willing. RA is tough, severe at times; but with a positive mind and action it can be managed and lived with. The journey continues.

Darragh Burke

Back in the day (the eighties and nineties, in other words) I was a very fit and active person playing any sport that I could; inter-county football for Wicklow, rugby in Naas and hurling with Hollywood, Co. Wicklow, my local club since I was old enough to kick a ball or hit a sliotar.

I started a trade as a carpenter/joiner after my leaving cert and also worked with my uncle, who was a local builder, doing whatever had to be done. My parents had a small family farm where we all helped out.

In January 1999, I picked up an injury, playing football for Wicklow, that bothered me for a couple of months and ruled me out of club games. I went to see the doctor that July with sore hands and after my examination I was started on an anti-inflammatory.

Returning to the GP two weeks later, I was given a referral letter to see someone in St Vincent's hospital, where I was diagnosed with RA.

Within a matter of weeks, my health was going downhill at a rapid pace.

I thought rheumatoid arthritis was a condition that only old people got and I knew very little about it.

I was started on various tablet concoctions and none of them worked. By October, I was admitted to Harold's Cross

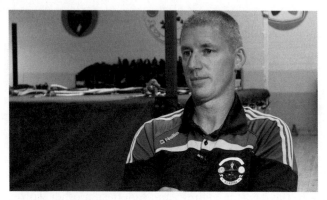

Darragh Burke

for rehab. I was now like a 100-year-old crooked man, unable to dress or undress myself properly, I couldn't bend down fully and all my joints were affected – from my little toe to my jaw.

My life was changing – and I had no control over it.

I was just married a year to Louise, we had only moved in to our house, and we had two small boys, Conor and Evan.

Out of work and with a mortgage to pay, things were stressful, to say the least.

After a few weeks in rehab, I had improved and returned home, where my wife was coping with our baby boy and young son – and now me, who also became dependant on her for lots of different things.

The pain was bad, but manageable; the fatigue was uncontrollable and still is my biggest problem to date.

After the shock of all the changes in my life, we started to get on with it as best we could. My wife went back to work and I became a stay-at-home dad. Louise worked all the hours she could, both in work and at home; she was the one that got things done and never complained. I would have been lost without her.

Family and friends helped too, organising a local fundraiser, helped finished off work in our house, even everyday jobs, like cutting sticks and cutting the grass.

Lots of Sundays over the following months were spent by my mam and dad going to see various healers, seventh sons of seventh sons, hoping to find a cure for me. Despite taking some lovely concoctions, it was all to no avail.

I tried to keep involved in some shape or form with my sons as they started football in Hollywood, which I did as a selector and I also helped with their training, as they moved up through their different age groups.

After a few years, I gave up attending the specialists, as I didn't feel any huge improvement and I felt I wasn't being listened to. I stuck to my local GP, Brendan, and I took the decision to stop taking medication as well. Taking them had felt like a full-time hangover, 24/7. My GP helped me through bad flare-ups over the following years with steroids, when needed. I also tried healing (something I didn't believe in it), reflexology and Reiki.

Life at home moved along. Louise worked and worked, and I looked after our lads and the running of the house, even managing to learn how to cook (well beans on toast!).

Fatigue, fatigue, fatigue is the killer. On lots of occasions, Louise would come home to find me asleep on the couch, the lads' homework not done and no dinner made – but I couldn't do anything about it.

My sons would help where they could, putting on my socks and picking up things off the floor. Even simple everyday jobs like peeling spuds or hoovering were challenging.

Over the years, even though it was very hard to do, I tried to exercise in some shape or form on a daily, weekly or monthly basis, depending on how I felt. I took part in an eight-week study at Harold's Cross on how exercise affects people with arthritis, where I met other people of different ages and with different types of arthritis. This made a great difference to my everyday life, so I kept it up as much as I could and it was great to chat to other people with similar conditions and circumstances.

In 2007, I spent a term in Harold's Cross because my hip was giving me pain. A total hip replacement was recommended by a specialist which happened with two surgeries in 2009 and 2011. I agreed to go back on medication, this time in the form of a biological injection, which was another changing point in my life, where I finally started to feel a huge improvement with my arthritis. I still take this drug on a weekly basis.

So, with the lads getting older and computers becoming part of everyday life and homework, not knowing how to plug one in, I looked into a course that would cater for my physical needs and total lack of computer knowledge, which the National Learning Network, Naas delivered.

While it took some time, but with great tutors and lots of patience, I got the hang of computers and received my ECDL cert. A follow-on part of the course was employer-based training, which I completed in the months after recovering from my hip replacement.

A work placement was part of the EBT course and I started with a company called Consafe, outside Athy, Co. Kildare. It was so different to what I had worked at before, I didn't know if I liked it or not, but I didn't have a lot of choices with my condition.

So, after lots of mistakes, I found that I enjoyed the work and wasn't too bad at it either. That was 2013 and I'm still there today on a part-time basis. It helps to have a boss who understands that living with arthritis has lots of ups and downs.

There is light at the end of the tunnel. You don't travel this journey on your own. Family, friends, doctors, social workers, occupational therapists, physiotherapists, healers – they are all valuable companions on the road.

I might have arthritis, but arthritis doesn't have me.

Ken Byrne

Growing up, I played soccer with Home Farm; I was lucky enough to play on a team that was filled with gifted and brilliant players and together we went unbeaten for over seven years, 206 domestic matches, winning 197 of these and drawing the other nine. This was a Guinness World Record, one that will take some beating.

During this time, I was lucky to represent Ireland on nine occasions, I also went to England for a number of trails for some of the big clubs.

Football is a fickle sport and I just failed to reach the top, mainly due to bad luck with injuries, but that's the way it goes.

As I got older, I played in the League of Ireland and then I moved abroad to Jersey in the Channel Islands. I continued to be active over there, playing soccer, water polo and generally, really active.

When I came home and got married, settled down, my sporting life took a back seat and life took over. Work and family life filled my time.

It was during this time I started to notice that I was slowing up, getting up in the mornings was becoming a bit of an effort. I'd joke and say it was old age, but gradually I was getting more and more aches and pains.

I recall getting my ankles checked out, as I was starting

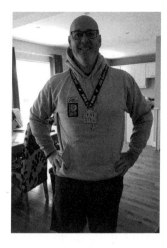

Ken Byrne

to struggle walking, it was becoming painful. The consultant mentioned that my cartilage was breaking up and it was this floating in my foot that was causing the issue. Then, casually, he mentioned he could see some arthritis in there too.

I didn't think much of it at the time and, to be honest, did nothing about it. I got surgery on my ankle to get the cartilage removed and that was that.

I continued to get slower and slower in the mornings getting out of bed, sore and achy, tired as the day wore on, and grumpy. I wasn't my usual self; wasn't really enjoying this life. I remember thinking, I am too young to feel this old and sore.

And then one morning, I woke up and I couldn't form a fist with my hands; neither of them, they were very sore, my fingers and joints were swollen. I went to my GP and he did some tests and put me on a dose of steroids.

This helped for a bit, until I needed to go back about three weeks later with the same issue. It wasn't just that my hands were sore, I was really tired, sluggish, wiped out.

I wasn't sure what was wrong, just that something was.

My test results from my first appointment came back negative for rheumatoid arthritis, so my GP was saying it was viral.

I later found out that a lot of the testing done by GPs for arthritis returns negative, so I don't know why they bother, to be honest. I got referred to a rheumatologist and he took one look at my hands and confirmed RA.

So, this was it? Thirty-five and I had arthritis. At least, it explained all the crap I was feeling; now, how to deal with it?

I was initially put on a DMARD (disease-modifying anti-rheumatic drug), which was strong and had a tonne of side effects, which I wasn't overly keen on, but it did start helping.

Over the years I was put onto other drugs too; a biologic which I injected twice a month for about two years, but then hit a plateaux where I really was not seeing any help or improvement. I was still sore and stiff.

Then one day in the hospital, after a routine blood check, the doctor noted my iron level was elevated and decided to do a test for hemochromatosis. The test took six months to come back. For some reason, bloods are sent to four or five different places and it just takes this long. Lo and behold, my results confirmed my levels were sky high. Another reason for my tiredness and aching.

As a result of this, I was taken off all my medication for RA and instead they took a pint of blood from me every week for a year. I started this in January 2013 and by October 2013, my levels were coming down, but more importantly, I was starting to feel a little better. I was starting to have energy again and with a few painkillers I was starting not to hurt as bad.

By January 2014, I was feeling that I could start back in a swimming pool, I was very overweight at this stage; close to eight or nine years of not doing anything sporty and this was eating me up.

I hated the way I was and what this disease was also doing to my head.

This is often an unmentioned feature of this disease, the depression and devastation it causes to your life. It's not just the physical aspect.

For years, I'd just pretend to be ok, but putting up with pain like this eats at you, destroys your confidence and the person you used to be.

So, to the swimming, I started back and was shocked at how unfit I was. I couldn't do one length; honestly my arms were on fire, I tried for two and was so sore. This was going to be a long journey.

Cutting a long story short, what I found through the swimming and the odd venture into the gym, was I really could feel a difference in my aches and pains. When I finished a session, I was much less sore than I would have imagined.

I thought like everyone else, that exercise with my symptoms was the last thing you would want to do; however, it's the opposite in fact.

I also started losing weight, which again can only be good for joints and the body. I started to cut out junk food and then one evening a friend mentioned he was in a triathlon club.

A lightbulb moment – I just thought, wow, if I could do this, how cool would that be. The sportsperson in me was reawakened. I now had a goal; I had something to train for.

I was going to be 40 that September, and most of my friends and kids even, only knew me to be fat and lazy; this ex-footballer who just keeps talking about what he used to do. My goal: Dublin City Triathlon in August, a week before my fortieth.

Let me tell you, everyone laughed at me when I told them, but for the first time in about 12 years, I was in a good positive place and I had a goal. Now at this point, I knew nothing about the triathlon, except it was swim, bike and run.

There were a few hurdles to get over.

The bike: I didn't own one, had not been on a bike since I was a teenager in fact.

The run: Since my surgery, my consultant had told me that I'd never run again. This had put a stop to my marathon exploits and running in general. And, my ankles really do hurt; it's bone-on-bone pain.

So, me being me, I signed up anyway. I got a road bike on the bike to work scheme and got the gear. Ah, the gear, the lovely lycra-clad fat dad I was. I would go out training and my kids wanted to know where, so they or their friends would not see me.

I learned about triathlons, I learned there were different distances. Sprint distance is a 750m swim, 20k bike and 5k run. Olympic distance (which is a normal tri) is a 1.5k swim, 40k bike and 10k run.

Then you move to the stupid distance of half ironman: 2k swim, 90k bike and 21k run. Full ironman distance: 3.9k swim, 180k bike and a bloody full marathon 41.2k run.

I trained, I started to feel really good and the exercise really was helping my RA.

I did my first sprint triathlon and, to be honest, it was just the maddest thing I ever did. I was so unprepared and not fit, but I got through it. The swim was ok, the bike was not too bad either, but the run was awful.

Two hundred metres into it, my lower back muscles were having none of it and just cramped up. While I did the run, mostly I walked. I had absolutely no run training done beforehand, thinking, sure, I've run all my life playing football, I'll be ok for 5k. No, absolutely not.

But I did it – and I was hooked. The adrenaline, the sense of achievement and also the internal competition, I could do better, swim quicker, bike faster and try to bloody run.

Mostly, I wasn't giving up, as I was really seeing improvements in my training, my body, my mind, my pain and, in general, my life.

I had stumbled onto something that gave me my life back.

I did another sprint in September and then decided that if I were to continue, I'd join a club and learn properly.

I joined Pulse Triathlon club a year later (when I was brave enough) and it was the best thing ever; I made so many new friends and just have fun and laughs every time.

Since joining, I have completed many more sprint distance triathlons, but I've done two Olympic distances and in 2017, I did Ironman 70.3 in Dublin. This was the biggest thing I'd ever done, it was massive. I did it in 8hrs 23 mins, a full seven minutes before the cut-off of eight-and-a-half hours.

In 2018, I signed up for the Dublin City Marathon. I decided it was now or never. I was also put on the waiting list for a new hip.

Again, me being me, I decided to put myself through months of sheer torture training with dodgy ankles and a hip that was getting worse as the weeks passed. I crossed the line in 6hrs 30mins – so so happy. I also managed three triathlons in 2018.

I got my hip operation in February 2019 and am in recovery, just back training, but clever training. I have more goals for the next two, three, four, years and I want to try to get my body into some sort of shape to allow me to try them.

I get emotional thinking how far I have come; believe me, it's not been easy, it's been filled with ups and downs, injuries, sickness, but would I change it? Not at all. Finding this road has given me my life back.

I get six weekly infusions now for inflammatory arthritis and still manage my hemochromatosis by getting a pint of blood taken about every two months. I struggle to balance my training with the days when I am exhausted and sore, it's a huge juggling act.

I also advocate for people to exercise who have autoimmune diseases, I blog and write about my journey. I want to keep it real for people with RA and other forms of this disease and inspire people not let it deter them. If you want something bad enough, there is always a way.

Maretta Byrne

As I write this, I'm still on the journey of having my rheumatoid arthritis controlled. My journey started with a pain in my back, or so I thought. In October 2018, at the age of 56 years, I was diagnosed with rheumatoid arthritis, so I'm a newbie!

From April/May 2018, I had a pain on the right-hand side of my back – not very specific. I took myself off to physio, took anti-inflammatories, but it was not going away. My physio did say that maybe it warranted an x-ray to see just what was going on. With summer looming, I said to myself, I will get around to that, as you do!

Coincidentally on a separate issue, I was due to have a steroid injection into my right shoulder in July. An ongoing problem for years. When I met with my orthopaedic consultant for the injection, my left shoulder was giving me a lot of pain and I asked would he mind injecting it rather than my right shoulder.

'Both shoulders; unusual,' he said. This was the first time the dots were beginning to join.

He asked if I had ever had a rheumatoid profile done. I knew I hadn't, as I didn't even know what he was talking about.

I was then referred to a rheumatologist and bloods were

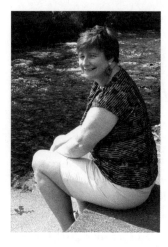

Maretta Byrne

taken by my GP. The results showed that I had elevated levels of rheumatoid factor in my blood. I also still had the pain in my back. Unknown to me at that time, this was the beginning of my RA journey.

My first visit with my rheumatologist was in September. He didn't confirm either way but wanted more bloods tests done, MRIs and generally to monitor how I was, before he could diagnose anything. He didn't seem too concerned about the pain in my back, as it was not a typical presentation of RA.

So, when I met with him a month later, I was not expecting a definitive diagnosis of rheumatoid arthritis – I even left my husband at home.

However, when he looked over my shoulder and asked was my husband with me – I knew!

This began the process of establishing exactly what RA was for me and where it was in my body – everywhere as it turned out! It transpires my shoulder pain, stiffness and restricted rotation in my neck and the pain in my back were all connected.

'Had I any other pain?' he asked. Was this the time to mention pains in my toes and my fingers? I couldn't recall if I had mentioned these pains to my GP; who goes to their GP saying they have a pain in their finger?

I very quickly realised that I had been carrying a lot of pain and self-medicating without seeing that they were all connected.

About 10 years ago, I was told I needed a hip replacement, but I kept going – this was in my control. I could decide to go to hospital and get it done when the pain was too bad and come home fixed! And that is exactly what happened.

But rheumatoid arthritis is different. I can't go into hospital and come home fixed. This is an autoimmune disease resulting in pains in all your joints.

The hardest things I find about rheumatoid arthritis, and they are in no particular order, are:
- It is out of my control,
- There is no cure for it,
- It is very painful,
- It is an invisible illness, and
- It is life-changing.

'Sure, it could be worse,' I would keep telling myself and others – but the counsellor in me would say 'This is my worse.'

As a counsellor/psychotherapist, I know acceptance is key. But I wasn't sure what it was I had to accept – all this pain?

I didn't know that each day I would have to 'check-in with myself'. How am I today? What can I manage to do today?

I continued to try to live my life as 'normal' – and anyone who knows me, knows I was very involved in everything and I was always running around doing something. But very quickly, my energy levels evaporated and my pain got worse.

I can now say that my life as I knew it changed overnight. My normal is now functioning at 50% capacity.

I was someone who walked an hour every day, now I can barely manage five minutes. A good friend said to me some time ago, what would it be like to admit you're struggling? And I guess that is key to acceptance.

The constant pain and fatigue, and I am not talking about the tiredness after a late night – it's waking up in the morning, with your head planning the day, but realising that as soon as I put my feet to the floor, that my body just isn't coming with me.

Anyone with RA will know exactly what I mean. This is fatigue like I never experienced before – and it's every day. Making plans to go out, looking forward to going, arriving and within the hour needing to come home, exhausted.

On a positive note, the medications and research into RA has advanced significantly in the last 10-15 years. So, once under control, I am told I will be able to resume a normal life. My treatment to date has involved a number of very strong medications, including a DMARD (disease-modifying anti-rheumatic drug), steriods and, more recently, infusions of a biologic.

One of the first line drugs given is a DMARD, which involves six tablets taken once weekly. I remember my consultant telling me to choose my day carefully as you need to be prepared to wipe out the next day!

So, now not only had I to deal with my RA, but I had a whole new set of woes to deal with – the side effects of the medication. I should say at this point, I didn't google rheumatoid arthritis. I guess I didn't want to know and I was in denial. I don't generally look at side effects of medications either!

But I do have side effects and, unfortunately, most days they feel worse than the condition itself.

Key to getting the RA under control is finding the right medication that works for you. The medications are very strong immune suppressors, so they come with lots of warnings. One of the DMARDs is a drug used in chemotherapy (albeit on a lower dose) – so headaches, nausea, fatigue, weight gain/loss, diarrhoea, are all part of the course and I am no exception.

For those days that my body is actually screaming out in pain (flare-ups) and the drug is just not hitting it, a course of steroids helps. Steroids are either your friend or foe. They are great for relieving pain, but for me play havoc with my overall physical and mental wellbeing – my foe!

I mentioned earlier that one of the hardest things was not having control over this disease, but another aspect which I find very hard is the fact that this is an invisible illness.

I never look sick and now I have gotten used to saying when asked, 'Ah, sure, don't I look great?' I have now stopped talking about 'it'.

I have always felt if I can look well on the outside, I might feel better on the inside! But all of this makes the illness even more invisible! I'm two people, what people see on the outside and what I am feeling in the inside.

There is no doubt this does have an impact on my mental wellbeing. As a psychotherapist, you'd think I'd have it all worked out – but that's not how it works.

It is a journey and there are plenty of bumps along the way. There are days when you physically can't do anything. Learning to sit and accept those days are part of the illness. As part of my own client work, I use an analogy of the 'jigsaw of life'. Each piece of the jigsaw is a part of your life – the challenge being that not one piece defines who you are.

If I look at my 'jigsaw of life' my RA is now a piece of this jigsaw. My challenge is to make sure that my arthritis is just a part of who I am and not let RA define who I am.

I am aware that key to living with RA means it is very important to get it under control. But this takes time and a lot of patience.

As I write this, I am eight months into this diagnosis and, unfortunately, it is still not under control. This means I am still in pain, quite stiff and the fatigue is ongoing; and I am also not sure what each day will bring.

On top of the DMARD, I have now started to have an infusion, which entails going in as a day patient to hospital once a month. If it works, the inconvenience of that will be worth it.

The hope is that eventually I can reduce the DMARD and as a result reduce my side effects.

The key to this diagnosis is acceptance. But it is very hard to accept when your body is still in pain – and that's the journey I'm on.

I have found that having a good support structure around me is so important. Not everyone needs to understand – but I now know that those closest to me need to be aware of what it is I am going through.

Jumping out of bed before they came home, pretending all is 'grand' may work for a while, but it eventually wore me down. I needed a place where I could just be myself, we all do. So, if a dinner was not on the table or they found me asleep in bed, I had to accept that that was okay. Letting my children in on what exactly was going on for me, gave me permission to 'be'.

However, for me, historically the go-to person, the strong one, admitting I was struggling was very hard. My husband and three boys keep me going every day and I try to keep going for them. I am so fortunate also to be surrounded by good friends who won't let me give up. As long as I keep making those 'plans' I guess I am still in some control.

As I continue on my journey with RA I keep in mind what my consultant said, 'We will get you to a point where the only indication that you have RA, will be the fact that you are taking medication.'

Wow, wouldn't that be great!

As I write, I hang onto this hope, while visualising the life I did have and not giving up on the hope that one day soon I will have it again.

In reading this story, it may seem a little depressing. But it's honest. I'm in the early stages of this diagnosis and, as such, learning to adjust to living with RA. If by writing this reflection on where I am at helps others starting out on their journey, then it's a good thing.

When I was diagnosed back in October, I knew no one or could find nowhere that gave me an honest indication of what lay ahead.

Zelda Carlyle

Mummy, it hurts! Circa 1980. I am eight years old.
Looking back now, this would have been the first
indication that all was not right. After many doctor visits,
my mum went with our family doctor's opinion that I was
suffering from growing pains. I had bouts of horrendous pain
in my arms and elbows, but nothing could be done to ease it.

Around the same time, my brother, who was seven years
older than me, was diagnosed with juvenile arthritis.

As time went on, the pain went away and it wasn't until
I had my first 'real' job in Smurfits that I began suffering
serious knee pain which landed me in the Blackrock Clinic
getting my knee drained.

The knee pain continued for the next few years, but only
to the extent that I needed to wear a knee support for sport.

Fast forward to the summer of 2011. I had given birth
to my third child in February and we headed off on a family
holiday to the sun in July. While we were away, the same knee
swelled up, but I didn't think too much of it.

After a long flight home, my knee was so swollen that I
couldn't bend my leg, so off I headed to A&E in the Beacon
Hospital where I was scheduled to have an arthroscopy.

Within a few days I was back on my feet with an
appointment to see the orthopaedic surgeon to get my results.

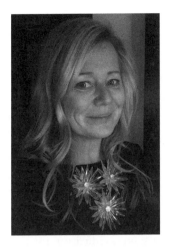

Zelda Carlyle

The results pointed to seronegative arthritis.

I was shocked. I was too young to have this old person's disease!

I was shown a list of rheumatologists' names and asked to pick one.

Within two days of being diagnosed, I was back in surgery having my knee drained again.

Over the next six months, my body went through the mill. My knees were being drained and injected every other week, I had carpal tunnel, every joint in my body hurt. The disease had taken hold of my body and I was riddled with pain and swelling.

This was all happening to me at a time in my life that I should have been enjoying having a new baby; but instead I was immobile and was on crutches and had to reach out for help, which I found difficult as I always liked to paddle my own canoe.

I felt my body was letting me down at a time I needed to be in my full health and my kids needed me.

I was going through a rollercoaster of emotions, but

ultimately came to the conclusion that things could be worse and hopefully things would get better.

Over time, my professor worked very closely with me to find the right medication for me. There were a lot of ups and downs but eventually we got it right. Every time one biologic medication failed, fortunately there was another to try.

One of the hardest things for me was all the comments about how well I looked and how could I really be as sick as I was making out.

RA is very much an invisible illness, but I have fought it hard and learned to live with the good days and the bad days.

Fortunately, I have been on the same medication for the last four years and it's still doing its job. I get the odd ache and pain, but I can definitely live with that.

Over the last nine months, I have had to have three surgeries, one of them a partial nephrectomy after being diagnosed with renal cancer. I have come out the other side cancer-free, so I feel very blessed that even though my body has broken down a few times, I've gotten back up each time.

I'm ready to live each day and be thankful that I have the love and support of my family and friends and that I have a great medical team that is looking after me.

I am also very aware that I am lucky to live in a time when biologic drugs are available, because I know without them, life would be very different. Having gone through cancer and serious surgery this year, I have realised that I may have RA, but RA doesn't have me – and it doesn't define me.

I will continue to have fun and defy my body.

Pamela Collins

I look well, but I'm not.

7am alarm goes off; very slowly I stretch every muscle in my body, sliding to the side of the bed, sitting up I feel it, looking in the mirror half amused at my bed head.

Then, here we go, standing up, I get that sinking feeling in my stomach as the pain starts in my feet, my ankles. They just don't want that pressure on them.

I walk to the window to open the blinds; when I say I walk, I mean my duck waddle!

At this point, my lower back has just woken up and has no intention of cooperating. Still doing my duck waddle around the bedroom, I reach for my morning meds, fumbling with tablet boxes, my stiff swelled sausage fingers drop the same tablet four times. This is just the first 15 minutes of my day and I already know and have acknowledged most of my joints as each one is like a stubborn two-year-old throwing a tantrum and not wanting any part in my day.

Standing at the top of the stairs, feet, ankles, knees complaining constantly, I look at these 14 steps and think I'm 37 years old and this stairs is my mountain every day.

Swelled achy fingers on the rail, not really trusting them; the complaining lower joints decide they are willing to half-participate in descending the stairs. Funny really, I never gave

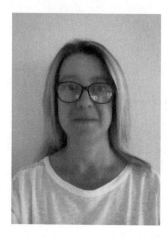

Pamela Collins

those stairs a bit of notice 10 years ago.

My duck waddle is slowly starting to change into a half-normal walk as I make some breakfast, trying to open a jar, reaching for my little helper to open the jar and again I think I'm 37 years old!

I finish up breakfast and start my physio stretches and then for my daily walk, my daily penance! I know I have to keep the physio going. I'm off, earphones in my ears, it's a nice morning.

I watch as people so full of energy head to work, college and it's been a long time since I've been able to work. Here I am, just walking and feeling every bit of it, and being overtaken by a woman twice my age!

I smile to myself as I get home, as I feel a sense of achievement after finishing my walk; my body still complaining, but also a little freer.

As I look at my watch, I realise I'm meeting the girls for shopping and some lunch, a rare treat for myself.

OH, DEAR LORD!! As I get ready, like any woman, oh I have nothing to wear, but I won't try on the 50 outfits.

My body won't allow that and I'd only waste my energy, so I settle on comfort (as always). I apply my make-up fighting and fumbling with lids and stiff, swelled fingers. Standing, I look in the mirror; smiling, I look well, but I don't feel it.

I meet my friends, all of whom have known me most my life. We hug and chat and then here it comes, 'Pam you look so well.' I'm delighted with the complement, but a wave of sadness comes, if they could really see how 'WELL' I am.

By the third shop, my lower back, knees, ankles have gone into a full-on screaming tantrum. Burning, severe pain, tiredness. Stubbornness kicks in and I mentally tell my body 'No, not today, I'm not missing out.'

Tears in my eyes, I think, 'Yeah, I look well,' and again the thought that I'm 37.

Sitting on the bench outside the shop, my dearest friend comes over and she knows, she simply smiles and says 'I've enough of shops, let's eat.'

Over lunch, I explain about my new meds or physio and the fact that my flare-ups aren't as bad as they used to be. In a soft tone, she says, 'Well you look so well.'

Yes, I do look well, but I'm not.

In 2010, I woke up like any other day, except on this day, I woke up in severe pain in most of my body, every joint in my body screaming, burning so hot I couldn't move.

I was terrified, no matter what I tried, the pain was unbearable.

I looked at my hands, I couldn't make a fist as my fingers were so stiff and swollen into sausages.

I was diagnosed with rheumatoid arthritis and osteoarthritis in my lower back. I also have Raynaud's disease, Graves' disease and localised myxedema.

It is difficult to see anything wrong with me, unless you

see my scars from the surgeries over the years, or if you see me in the mornings/early afternoon or when my body has gone into full flare-up mode.

If you look closely enough, you will see that I will always walk a bit funny and slower, that I fumble at check-outs with change.

If I bend down to pick something up, I might stay down there for a while, not because I like the scenery, but because my lower back has decided it's gone on a break.

I might greet you with a smile or hug, but don't take offence if I don't shake hands with you, as it kills my already stiff fingers if someone grips them too tightly.

During a conversation, don't worry I'm still listening, I just can't sit that long. I haven't gone off you and I know we made plans and this is the second or third time I've cancelled, but you see my body has a completely different diary of its own and it only informs me at the last minute what our day is going to be.

This is just a mix of what my day can be like since being diagnosed with RA. I have learned so much about myself and that, yes, I have a chronic condition that can change you and your life, but it can be managed and with good management and self-awareness, you can live a normal life, normal for you, a person with RA.

Jennifer Conlan

Rheumatoid arthritis is the name given to just one disease, although no two individuals affected by it will experience it in quite the same way. Each person affected by this autoimmune disease has had their life altered dramatically; from home-life to work-life, from relationships to friendships.

My RA story will share some similarities with others, but from my own slightly different perspective. I was a happy, healthy, busy young doctor until I was struck down with this debilitating disease that I had only previously studied in medical school and had observed in patients. I never dreamt that one day I would become the patient rather than the doctor.

I had a naïve perception that doctors were invincible, they never got sick but rather treated those that were and surely if they ever did become ill, they could just make themselves better again!

Well, I learnt the hard way that doctors are just like everybody else and unfortunately just as susceptible to disease and sickness. Despite my medical background it was not a straightforward process finding a diagnosis to explain my early symptoms. This proved to be a long and frustrating road for me and I will therefore tell my story in two parts; pre- and post-diagnosis.

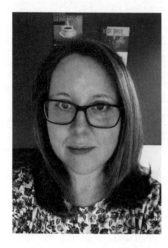

Jennifer Conlan

Pre-diagnosis

I am not too sure when my RA story should begin, but I believe it may have started around 12 years ago, when I was a medical student. My right index finger became swollen for no apparent reason and I couldn't bend it at all. I went to my GP and she diagnosed tendonitis in my finger, but noted that my blood tests revealed a positive rheumatoid factor.

She was not overly concerned about that though, as rheumatoid factor can be raised in people with no underlying condition. I have since learned that a swollen finger can be a common early presentation of rheumatoid arthritis and is usually followed by a long symptom-free period.

Around the same time, I also began to suffer from fatigue, which I put down to the gruelling schedule in medical school and the long hours spent studying. Looking back though, I seemed to struggle somewhat more than my peers. I don't particularly recall suffering from any pain at that time and it was a number of years later when my pain began to gradually creep in.

In the early years of my career as a junior doctor I was

frequently unwell, mainly with respiratory tract infections, and suffered both mentally and physically due to the punishing shifts I was working. I appeared, once again, to struggle more than others in my position, but despite many doctor visits I couldn't quite put my finger on what the problem was.

The pain started gradually, but only flared-up a few days before 'that time of the month'. It was an aching 'flu-like' pain that I could feel all over my body, in my joints and in my muscles. The moment my period started all of the pain would instantly go away again. I thought this was odd, but ignored it for a while and the aches and pains almost came as a surprise to me each month until I started to notice there was a pattern.

More doctor visits later and it just seemed like a premenstrual syndrome (PMS) symptom and I started taking prescribed painkillers from around the middle of my cycle in preparation for this inevitable pain phenomenon I was afflicted with each month.

It went on like this until I was pregnant with my first child. I came off the painkillers and I experienced the usual painful niggles of pregnancy, but my typical aches and pains ceased for the duration of the pregnancy. After my son, Dylan, was born the pain returned and once again I was commenced on painkillers. I was so disappointed because I had almost forgotten about this mystery pain during the nine months of my pregnancy.

The real problems began after the birth of my daughter, Emma, two years later. Once again, I was pain-free during the pregnancy with the exception of the usual pregnancy-related pains. When Emma was born the pain came back again within a couple of months, except that this time it was worse than ever and accompanied by a crippling fatigue like none I had experienced before.

I began to notice some changes in my fingers and the pain specifically affected my joints more than before. After a bit of research, I began to suspect I could have rheumatoid arthritis. I confided in my parents and learned that rheumatoid arthritis was indeed on my dad's side of the family, including young onset-RA.

I discussed my concerns with my GP and was referred to a rheumatologist in the Mater Private Hospital in Dublin. That first consultation was life-changing.

I left with a diagnosis of RA, confirming my suspicions, and validating how I had felt for so long up until this point. I left with a prescription in my hand for a DMARD (disease-modifying anti-rheumatic drug) and folic acid, a treatment regime most newly diagnosed RA patients are commenced on.

The consultant was wonderful and, far from being upset with the diagnosis, I was relieved to finally have a name to put to what I had been feeling for years. It wasn't all in my head and I wasn't completely crazy after all!

The pain I had experienced each month before my period was a flare-up of the RA. The pain went away during my pregnancies as the RA went into remission, which is quite typical for this condition. The pieces of the puzzle were finally fitting together.

My husband, family and friends were so supportive and it felt good to know that everyone finally understood how I had been feeling for so long.

I was 36 years old when I was diagnosed, roughly 10 years after my initial symptoms began. It had been a long journey to get to that point.

I had studied rheumatology in medical school during this time, but RA was only on my radar as an illness that affected others. I had had the privilege of examining patients with rheumatoid arthritis and taking their medical histories as a student. They were all elderly people, so it was ingrained in me that this was a condition affecting older people.

I was particularly interested in 'rheumatoid hands' as this regularly came up in short case examinations in the finals! I knew all about features such as swan neck deformities, Z-thumbs and Boutonniere deformity. It affected many joints in a symmetrical pattern in the body. It caused fatigue and didn't just affect the joints, but also many of the organ systems. I could list off the signs and symptoms and knew all about the available treatments and their side effects.

Despite all of this knowledge and knowing that RA can affect all ages, even young children, it was difficult to come around to thinking that this was what I had all along, that a young person like me could have rheumatoid arthritis. It is certainly not an obvious or easy diagnosis as I had once believed. I had only ever seen patients with advanced disease and 'typical features' of a generation that unfortunately didn't have the effective treatments available to us today.

Rheumatoid arthritis is not easy to diagnose and it can take years to be diagnosed and treated, by which time some irreversible damage has already likely occurred.

I also realised that the knowledge of the disease from medical textbooks and meeting with patients afflicted with RA did not give me a full understanding of what it is truly like to live with rheumatoid arthritis. Unfortunately, I had to learn that by experiencing it the hard way, by living life with rheumatoid arthritis.

Post-diagnosis
The DMARD seemed to improve my symptoms initially, but unfortunately it wasn't a wonder drug for me and in the two

years since my diagnosis I have progressed through a number of medications including biologics. The wonder drug that will make all of my pain and struggles go away unfortunately still eludes me.

There are more medication options available, so I try not to lose hope that I will eventually start a medication that works for me and achieves a remission of my RA.

Instead, I have adapted to my condition as best I can, with various kitchen gadgets, grooming aids and even an automatic car. I try to accept my limitations, especially during particularly bad flare-ups, and more importantly to forgive myself for what I just can't do day-to-day. I regularly feel guilty for not being able to run around with the kids or get down on the floor to make that jigsaw puzzle or for allowing them to watch a little bit too much TV when I just have to lie down and take a nap.

I have not been well enough to work for quite a while now. Only time will tell if and when I can return to my job as a medical lecturer. I experience financial worries and the medical expenses add to this worry, but it's just another situation I have had to adapt to and manage in the best way that I can. It has been a huge life change to go from career woman to 'stay-at-home mom' with a chronic health issue. However, I look on it as a positive thing that I can at least spend more time with the kids than I would have otherwise. For now, it is an accomplishment to get the kids to and from school and just look after them.

When I was first diagnosed, there was indeed a sense of relief, but I was also terrified to think that I had this lifelong illness and would require some serious medication to control it. I was already prone to respiratory tract infections, so I was concerned about taking medications that dampen the immune response and would leave me even more prone to infections.

I had a great-grandmother who spent a great deal of her life in hospital due to rheumatoid arthritis, so I couldn't help but fear that this was a fate that could also befall me. It didn't seem fair to have a diagnosis like this at such a young age and I felt isolated as I didn't know anyone else with RA. I didn't know where to turn until one day I discovered a group on Facebook specifically for people in Ireland with rheumatoid arthritis under the age of fifty. I joined the group and this has been a lifeline for me. It is wonderful to know that I am not alone and that I have others to talk to who can truly understand what I am going through.

Arthritis Ireland organise plenty of events throughout the year and I have attended some talks and even a conference for people under 50 with RA. Events such as these provide opportunities to meet face-to-face with others like myself and also to learn of new advances in RA research. I have gotten many tips about managing the condition as well as meeting lots of great people.

It's a tough road I'm on, but there is great comfort in knowing that I am not travelling it alone, that others with rheumatoid arthritis will be there for me and that I can be there for them.

My RA story is just one of many with lots of similarities, whilst no two stories will be exactly the same. I hope that by telling my story that others will find comfort in knowing that they are not alone with this illness. Finally, I may have rheumatoid arthritis, but rheumatoid arthritis does not have me! It has greatly impacted my life, but RA does not and will not define who I am.

Noeleen Conway

This is my story.

I was 18 when I was diagnosed with RA; I am now 40 years old. I wasn't long out of secondary school, working as a waitress in a local pub. In the bath one night, I could see that both of my knees looked swollen; from what I can remember I had no other signs or pain.

I went to my GP and he got me to walk across the room and after examining me, he diagnosed me there and then with arthritis. He was an amazing doctor; I was so lucky to have such a brilliant doctor, he really helped me with everything I went through.

The diagnosis affected my parents more than me. I was born with dislocated hips and was lying face down on a frame for the first 12 weeks of my life. My parents still blame that, but it wasn't their fault; they just did what the doctors told them to do.

I would let on to them that I was fine, but I was crippled as it got worse; I could see how it affected them and tried to hide it from them.

Referred to Dún Laoghaire for x-rays, I remember seeing people with one leg, people in wheelchairs, and thinking that I was lucky, it could be so much worse.

I started getting fluid drained from my knees, was getting

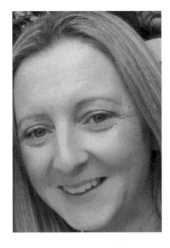

Noeleen Conway

steroid injections and had an arthroscopy done in St Vincent's. I was on anti-inflammatories, a DMARD (disease-modifying anti-rheumatic drug) and then biologics after switching consultants.

They didn't work for me, however, and things were getting worse, it was now in my hips. Travelling to Dublin every day for work was getting harder. I remember holding on to the wall sometimes for support walking down the street, and my friend would link me if we went out for lunch. Eventually, I was not fit for work.

I was on steroids more than I was off them. A night out, a party, our wedding and honeymoon – steroids helped get me through.

Eventually, my consultant in Clane sent me to Blanchardstown, where I was started on a great biologic treatment, which was really working for me. But I was getting to the stage where I wanted to start a family, which meant coming off the treatment before even trying, so I did.

After two months, I could hardly walk and had to go back on the drug, but this time it didn't work for me.

I just thought we would never have children, which was very hard for me as most of my friends were starting families. It was a really low time for me.

My husband was brilliant, he told me he married me for me, he was such a great support to me during it all.

I cried for the first time in with my doctor, who told me that I needed a hip replacement. They were putting it off, because of my age and trying different treatments.

I had my first hip replacement in February 2010, which was a turning point for me. I had a new life. I could walk again, without feeling like my hip was going to break.

After being off work for five years, in May 2011, I was deemed fit for work again. I was so lucky to still have my job after so many years. Going back to work put having a baby out of my head.

My doctor was thinking differently though and the last time I saw him before returning to work he said, 'Hopefully, the next time I see you, you will be pregnant.'

Two months later, five pregnancy tests and another one in the GP clinic just to be 100% sure, yes, I was pregnant. We told my parents straight away; it was the best news ever.

I flew through my pregnancy, no pain, and Sean arrived in March 2012 by c-section; 8lbs 12 ozs of joy that we thought we would never have. He was and still is perfect.

But six weeks after having Sean, my arthritis came back and I went back on treatment. Then in May 2013 I had my other hip done. This was harder, as I was leaving Sean at home and couldn't lift him, or have him on my knee for six weeks, but we laid on the bed for cuddles.

So, all was great again, I was back working full-time, then I had a miscarriage in February 2016. It was heart breaking, but we were lucky enough to have Sean to go home to. I was turning 38 that year, so I decided if I didn't get pregnant again before December, we would be thankful to have Sean.

In early December 2016, we found out that I was pregnant again and everything was perfect this time. Ciara arrived on 2 August 2017 by c-section, 10lbs 11ozs of perfection. This pregnancy was harder though, with a lot of lower back pain, and again the arthritis came back six weeks after having Ciara.

After all the years of pain and thinking we couldn't even try to start a family, we now have two beautiful children. I am working and my pain is being managed, after having two hip replacements and a biologic infusion every four weeks in Blanchardstown.

To my husband, my parents, my family, friends, Dr Moloney, Dr Barry, Mr Paddy Kenny – thank you. I wouldn't have got through it all without you.

To anyone who is suffering and can relate to my story, try to stay positive and never give up. As my father always said, it will all work out in the end – and it does.

Petraea Costello

My story begins with a struggle to open a shampoo bottle. It begins with an inability to tie my hair back. Crying in the shower wondering why my fingers won't work? Where did this stiffness come from all of a sudden?

My RA story begins with a visit to the GP, who confirmed I had the rheumatoid factor, elevated CRP and ESR. What are these acronyms? What are they on about? I am a fit and healthy 21-year-old. This doesn't happen to someone like me. I am young.

My story begins with tears streaming down my face, head held in my hands, sitting on a park bench outside the Blackrock Clinic, where the specialist uttered those words you never want to hear, 'You have rheumatoid arthritis.'

The sadness, anger and bitterness grabbed me all at once. I had to make that dreaded phone call to tell my mam and boyfriend through tears. It was hard to articulate the words 'rheumatoid arthritis'. And I have hated those words ever since. That was 20 years ago.

This is now. 41 years old, married, two kids, living back in the west of Ireland after a long stint living abroad. To look at me, you'd think there was nothing wrong. I go to the gym. I am fit and healthy.

But people don't see the tears and pain. They don't see

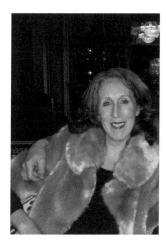

Petraea Costello

you staring at the ceiling at 5am in the morning wondering how you are going to get going. You pop a painkiller and hope for the best. You limber up throughout the day and you feel a little better. The excruciating morning stiffness has gone. You're left with a milder pain in your hands, shoulders and knees. But you can cope with that. Until it starts again the next morning when you stare at that ceiling all over again.

It's hasn't all been bleak. I have been very lucky. The journey of someone living with RA is usually akin to being on a roller coaster. There are good months and years, and then there are the not so good times.

When flare-ups take over your life. When the disease consumes you every day. When that's all you think about. And you hate the fact that it's winning. I've had many great years when the disease was well controlled with one of the oldest drugs on the market.

My rheumatologists in Dubai and Sydney said I was lucky. I never realised until now how lucky I was back then.

Then there were dark years for sure when I was trying to conceive in my early 30s.

For me, when the drug is working and there is no pain or inflammation, you forget you almost have the disease and go into this false sense of security. You don't think you actually need the drug at all. That you are grand! Then you go off your drug. And then you realise you were wrong. You do need those drugs. They are controlling you after all.

It took longer to conceive and it was tough, but I got there in the end. Pregnancy dampens the disease for some reason, so you get a 'break'. But it rears its ugly head again about six weeks after giving birth and you are back to square one.

Then you start to explore all the alternative therapies. You read endless articles about miracle cures. You listen to the podcasts. You try supplements. You try more supplements. You'd be a very rich woman if you got a cent for every time someone said to you 'Have you tried turmeric?' You go to acupuncturists, you do moxa, essential oils, Emotional Freedom Therapy tapping, accuenergitics, functional medicine, drink apple cider vinegar, do food intolerance testing and kinesiology.

But when the drugs are working, you are ok. You do fine. You function. You can exercise and do the things you want to do. So, you aren't looking for an answer because the drugs are the answer. They are working for you. And although you hate the idea of being on drugs for the rest of your life, the benefit outweighs the risks. That's what you think. That's what you try to believe, but deep down you are scared of the effects and toll the drugs are having on your body. And you know that your periodontal disease isn't a coincidence either. That if you have one autoimmune disease, you usually get another. Great.

Then you move back to Ireland and things turn bleak

again. The drugs stop working. One day you go back to struggling to open the shampoo bottle. So, you try other drugs. You look for answers. You are waiting for that new hi-tech drug to work. It doesn't, so you move onto another hi-tech drug and that doesn't work either.

Your rheumatologist says there are endless options, so you live in hope. And you wait. Wait for the morning that you don't feel pain. You are sad, angry and bitter again. So, you go off gluten. You quit dairy. You quit meat. You avoid tomatoes and some nightshades. You want an answer. A solution to the problem. You are waiting to see whether that's the answer. It's very early days, but I'm still waiting…

But you never stop wondering, where did I get this from? Why me? I am hopeful. I don't want this nasty disease to beat me. To control me. I will find a way.

Ann-Marie Costello/McHale

My first experience of rheumatoid arthritis was at the age of 33. I had just given birth to our first child. My husband and I had relocated to Hong Kong 12 months earlier and I was missing the presence of extended family and friends on occasions like this.

Within two weeks of giving birth, the knuckles of my right hand became suddenly inflamed and very sore. I struggled to fasten the little studs of my new-born's babygro. When I squeezed the studs between my finger and thumb the pain would dart up both fingers making that simple task almost impossible. One particular day I remember thinking that if this pain continued, I would be in a wheelchair by the time I was 40. These thoughts – combined with the trauma of childbirth and caring for my newborn baby – left me feeling very low and frightened.

I had no idea why my knuckles were sore, red and swollen, or why I was feeling continously tired and unable to cope when previously I had been full of energy. I recall running the cold tap on my fingers in an attempt to get some temporary relief. At first, the pain and swelling were confined to the fingers of my right hand, but soon the pain extended to the toes on my left foot.

Living in Asia, the obvious first port of call for me was to

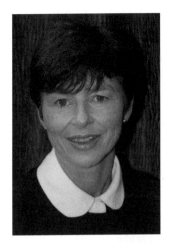

Ann-Marie Costello/McHale

try alternative medicine. Here I was diagnosed with adrenal gland burnout and prescribed lots of supplements including B12 and a form of steroid. After six-eight months on these treatments and with no improvement, I was then diagnosed with mercury poisoning and advised to have all my silver fillings removed and replaced with white fillings ... which I duly did.

This procedure made no difference to my health. If anything, the removal of the fillings put further strain on me physically and emotionally.

After 18 months of alternative medical remedies and still no improvement to my health, I decided to pursue the conventional medical route and made an appointment with my GP.

He confirmed a diagnosis of rheumatoid arthritis very quickly. For me, this was relatively good news as I now had a concrete diagnosis. It also came as no great shock as I had read that the risk of sudden onset RA is increased after childbirth in women who are prone to it.

The GP started me on a course of anti-inflammatories

and then I progressed to stronger medications working right up to a DMARD (disease-modifying anti-rheumatic drug) which caused allergic reactions. In the meantime, I became pregnant with our second child, so my need for medication was eliminated as I was in remission for nine months.

However, after that pregnancy I had a major flare-up, which apparently is the norm. It was at this stage also that we returned to Ireland.

I then decided to start a new care plan and consulted a rheumatologist. After extensive examinations and x-rays he prescribed what was then a relatively new biologic treatment, which is administered by injection weekly.

I have been taking this biologic weekly since 2006 and with great success. I have blood tests every six months to check for the presence of TB, which is a side effect sometimes associated with this medication. Thankfully, it has worked for me and without any major side effects to date.

In recent years – and in consultation with my rheumatologist – I tried to reduce the dosage to every other week, but I experienced flare-ups of the condition and so reverted back to the weekly dose.

I still get painful episodes after physical work, especially in the major joints like my hips. In addition, joints that have old injuries become painful after a lot of exercise.

My father had rheumatoid arthritis from his early forties onwards, and my memory is of him having to come in from the farm and go to bed in the afternoon, such was his pain and exhaustion. While he experienced many RA symptoms, he tested negative in the rheumatoid factor blood test. This is also true in my own case.

It is often forgotten that, as well as the pain, symptoms such as exhaustion, lack of energy, depression – and for some people low levels of fever – are all symptoms of RA. Thankfully, I don't experience all these symptoms during a flare-up, but I do need to keep in mind that these other symptoms go hand-in-hand with this condition.

I am now 51 years old and lead an active life. I work full-time, try to swim a couple of times a week and do the occasional 8k run with my teenage daughter; yes, that's the baby that I could hardly dress 18 years ago.

Niamh Coughlan

I'm a 19-year-old student from Cork, currently studying for an undergraduate degree in UCC. To get where I am today was not easy and I would like to share my story with you.

My story begins in May 2013 when I was aged 13. I had just come to the end of my first year in secondary school. In the months prior to this, I had been experiencing slight pains in my hands and feet. I loved sport and played a lot of camogie and Gaelic football with both school and club teams, and thought the pain was a sport-related injury.

My first set of summer exams were just completed when the pains in my hands began to get worse. My mum made an appointment to see the GP and I had my diagnosis by the end of that week.

I can clearly remember my eyes filling with tears hearing the doctor tell me that I would have to take some time off from playing sport and that any form of contact sport was not recommended. I was told that I had juvenile arthritis, but more tests were to be done to determine which type exactly. With this, I was also diagnosed with Raynaud's phenomenon, a condition which affects the blood vessels.

I could not comprehend how a person my age could have arthritis. Being a child, I had always associated it with older people. Part of me doubted the doctor as I did not want to

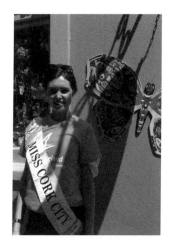

Niamh Coughlan

believe that I had anything like this and I began doing my own research, wanting to prove it was something else.

At the time I was about 5'11" (I've always been tall) and so I thought I had just been going through a phase of growing pains. I was prescribed short-term steroids to calm the inflammation and I was referred onto a children's consultant in the CUH.

It was a few weeks before I was seen, but an overview of my entire body confirmed that this was in fact a form of arthritis.

In the following months, the pains got worse, I was experiencing stiffness in the mornings. There were even tears before school sometimes, as simple tasks like doing the buttons on my shirt became a challenge.

I began to do my own research on what causes the disease and how to get rid of it, but I was told prevention from further damage was the main thing to be concerned about.

I went from playing on the pitch to watching from the sideline, which really affected my overall mood, as sport was a great outlet for me to have fun and keep fit.

School life got harder too, as I soon noticed my hand would get sore after a short time from writing, as well as experiencing knee pain from carrying the weight of heavy books around all day. I had tried hand supports and occupational therapy, but nothing really relieved the burning sensation and swollen joints. It also began to impact my social life with friends, as I was lethargic and conscious of my condition.

A few months later I was transferred to the children's rheumatology department in Our Lady's Children's Hospital in Crumlin. The doctors there were specifically focused on arthritis in children, so I had hope that they would be able to solve it. They went through possible solutions and explained to me that the main aim was to prevent the arthritis from getting any worse, and that long-term medication was the best solution.

They introduced me to a commonly used disease-modifying drug (DMARD), which I would self-inject once a week. I remember crying through the whole appointment as I listened to what could potentially happen if I did not try something before it got any worse. Personally, I am not so keen on taking anything as I like to allow the body to repair itself, so agreeing to trying this was not easy for me.

The following week a nurse came to my house to demonstrate to me how to use the drug. I learned about the side effects and agreed that a Friday would be best to take it as I wouldn't have school the day after.

The next nine months were horrible. I was sick every Friday night and Saturday, and by the time Monday morning came around I was extremely tired. There wasn't a huge improvement in how I was feeling and, in the mean time, the pain had moved to both joints in my jaw. My entire face would swell and I had trouble sleeping at night due to the constant clicking of joints in and out of place. I was diagnosed with TMD (temporomandibular disorder) which affects the jaw joint and facial muscles. I got steroid injections into both sides of my jaw and also in my fingers with the hope that these would ease things.

It wasn't long before I was referred on to a professor in CUH who specialises in this area. Thankfully during these few months, I met with members from iCAN (the Irish Children's Arthritis Network) which was great, as I got to meet with other teenagers my own age who were also experiencing similar pain. This network does exceptional work for young children and teenagers who need support and they provide a platform in which these needs are met.

The following April, I met with the doctors again and I told them I would not continue to take the medication. My diagnosis was now described as a form of rheumatoid arthritis, but also enthesitis-related arthritis which specifically affects the ligaments surrounding the joints.

They wanted to try out a different medication, which still was an injection, but would not have the same side effects. I agreed to try it out and a month later I was changed to another medication which I continued to take for a while.

By this stage I was used to using the self-inject method and so I had no problems with doing it myself. The side effects were not as bad, but I was experiencing weight loss and hair loss, while searching for alternative methods to try to cure myself.

These symptoms especially affected my confidence and even my mental health began to suffer. I excluded myself from friends and I didn't like being in school. I stopped eating properly which only made problems worse. I ended up in hospital for a week the summer before my leaving cert, as I had lost nearly three stone in weight over a very short period of time. I felt helpless and that my life would continue the way it was going.

Although it has taken quite some time, I am almost back to the person I was before any of this had happened.

In 2017, I turned 18 and I was transferred back to Cork to the adult clinic in the CUH. I was still taking the biologic, at the time. I discussed with my doctors about coming off it, but was strongly advised to keep taking it, at least until the exams were over.

I went against my consultant's advice and stopped taking the medications four months before the leaving cert. I knew I was taking a big risk, as I had no idea how my body would react, but I was confident in my decision.

I am a driven person who always wants to achieve high, so I worked hard over the next few weeks. Thankfully everything seemed to be ok and I sat my exams with the help of a scribe which was a huge benefit to me. I was delighted with my results and am now studying French and art history in UCC; a four-year degree where I will spend third year studying in France.

As for today, I am now in a place where I can manage my symptoms. I don't like the cold as it seems to cause flare-ups in my hands and in my feet, but I've learned how to deal with difficult situations. I am currently medication-free and my symptoms have thankfully eased, apart from the odd day when I might get swelling in my hands.

Since starting college, I have slowly introduced myself to moderate exercise both outdoors and in the gym and it has definitely helped my symptoms ease. Earlier this year, I signed up to do the Vhi Women's Mini Marathon in Dublin in aid of Arthritis Ireland and I am proud to be raising money for a cause so close to my heart. The marathon took place on 2 June and I was delighted to have completed the run in just over an hour. The atmosphere on the day was incredible and I will definitely be returning to run again next year.

Earlier this year, I also entered Miss Cork and I was placed first runner-up in the competition, meaning I went forward to the semi-finals of Miss Ireland in July.

My experiences have given me an understanding of both the personal and social struggles with coping with this disease, but there are ways for everyone to become comfortable and confident in how they deal with their conditions. It just takes time!

Annette Dillon

They say life begins at forty, but for me just after my fortieth birthday, I woke up with pain in my knuckles on both hands. It was a very strange sensation, as my hands were also quite swollen and very sore.

At first, my reaction was just to see how things would go, maybe it would disappear as quickly as it had occurred. But obviously the symptoms didn't disappear; in fact, every morning my knuckles would be very painful, although it would ease slightly as the day went on. Also, I was feeling very tired.

At this time in my life, it was pretty busy, happily married with three children aged 15, 12 and 10, two girls and a boy, just doing the normal family things, looking after the home and everything that goes with it. There was one difference in our family, as our youngest child had been diagnosed with severe autism at quite an early age.

Having a child with a special need brings a lot of pressure and challenges onto a family, sometimes you feel you are coping well, trying your best; but our bodies sometimes have a way of letting us know that's not the case.

When my symptoms didn't seem to be improving, it was time to investigate a little more. This was scary, as usually we think the worst possible thing is happening to us, our minds

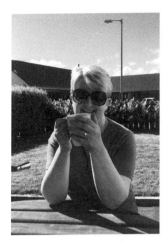

Annette Dillon

run wild with all that could be wrong.

Walking into the doctor's surgery that morning, I felt very nervous, wondering if I was wasting his time, would he think I was imagining these symptoms. Maybe leave it another couple of weeks to see if I would feel any better?

Once I was in the doctor's surgery, however, all that changed in an instant.

He took both my hands in his and began to examine each of my fingers separately. As soon as he touched my knuckles, the pain was very visible to him. After a full examination of my knees, elbows, feet and shoulders, he sat me down and explained that he needed me to have blood tests done.

Then he said he was nearly sure that I had rheumatoid arthritis, an autoimmune disease where the immune system attacks healthy tissues and joints in the body. Of course, most people when they here arthritis think of elderly people, so I was shocked to hear age doesn't really matter; in fact, you can be diagnosed at any age. Children can develop arthritis, which came as a huge surprise to me.

After another couple of weeks when the results of the

blood tests and x-rays came through, the diagnosis confirmed early stages of RA.

It was a relief that finally I knew what was going on, although naturally it was a very worrying time wondering what this all meant. Some people close to me were very shocked and upset, they probably had me written off straight away. My initial thought was it could be treated and managed, so I felt maybe I would cope, it was just another challenge sent my way.

It took a while before I finally got on the right road for me, I was put on steroids first, which were to attack the disease full-on, but I had a lot of uncomfortable side effects. Eventually, after attending the rheumatology unit at Our Lady's Hospital, Manorhamilton my experience began to turn around.

Under a rheumatology consultant everything about the condition was explained very clearly to me, including what can cause it. In my case a stressful incident such as learning that my youngest child had special needs could have been the trigger, although I have since discovered that it can also be hereditary. There are some relations in my family with RA also.

It has been nearly 15 years since my first diagnosis. For the past 10 years I have been taking a DMARD (disease-modifying anti-rheumatic drug) every Monday, followed by folic acid on Tuesday. This medication has been very successful for me. I realise that this medication doesn't always work for everyone, most people have their own story as to what works for them.

Rheumatoid arthritis is to me quite a silent disability. Unless you know the person has RA, sometimes you just couldn't tell. For me, life goes on as normal, you learn to cope with the condition. I have found a lot of help through Arthritis Ireland and whenever I had questions, my consultant and nurses have also been very important in managing my condition.

There are times of flare-ups when your arthritis becomes much more inflamed; you're tired a lot of the time, in my case, pains can suddenly appear in my knees, shoulders and always in my hands and wrists. Usually for me, this occurs on both sides of my body, and it is always a lot worse for me first thing in the morning.

I have noticed that if I am worried or stressed over anything, then it could bring on a flare-up, so I try to manage this with relaxation, yoga and meditation. Exercise is also very important for anyone dealing with RA.

It is very important that we find ways to deal with our own RA, of course this can be very different for everyone. Some days you won't feel like exercising, that is fine, do not feel guilty. There will be plenty of days when you will feel like moving about more. Listen to your own body it knows best.

Naturally, diet is very important. Having a balanced, healthy lifestyle will also benefit your RA. It's very important to educate yourself about the foods which are suited and beneficial.

Lastly, try to surround yourself with positive people who will listen when you're not feeling very well. This can be difficult, because it's not a visible disability and can go unnoticed. It's up people like us who live with RA to educate our families and everyone else.

Rheumatoid arthritis is a life-long condition. You will have good days and bad ones, but with the right management and a good team around you, it can also turn out to be positive, as I have experienced.

Sandra Fitzgerald

L iar liar pants on fire.
'How are you?' 'Great thanks.'
'Did you sleep ok?' 'Yes thanks.'
'Did you get here ok?' 'Yes, thank you, no problems.'
Liar.

Because the truth is:
How am I? Honestly, the fatigue is so bad I could lie down on this footpath right now and be asleep in seconds. The stabbing pain in my hip is so bad it's taking all my energy not to cry in front of you and the ache in my hands is so distracting I can barely follow our conversation.

Did I sleep ok? Well, once the sedatives kicked in, I was out like a light. If I didn't take them, I wouldn't sleep, they numb all the pain you see, so I get a kind of drunken slumber, but when I wake, I still feel like I didn't sleep at all. But up I get and off I go.

Did you get here ok? Just about, my ankles and knees locked up about 10 minutes ago when I reached my absolute limit of driving and my hands ache from holding the steering wheel. But I'm here now, I'll worry about the way home later.

This is my life now. It's easier to fake being well than to tell the truth. If I confessed to people how much I was actually struggling, I don't think I would have the relationships with people I have now. If I was honest about my struggles with rheumatoid arthritis, I think most people would just avoid me.

There's the people who think you are lying. 'You're too young to have arthritis.' I was diagnosed with rheumatoid arthritis at 24, but I get this one less now as I hurtle towards my forties. 'Who diagnosed you?' 'But how did they know it's arthritis?'

The people who ask, but really don't care; 'Sure we're all tired and sore, you're getting old.' To them I say just don't ask, my medical condition is none of your business anyway.

The 'helpful' people; gluten-free, sugar-free, dairy-free, sleeping upside down in a vat of cannabis oil (ok I made that one up) just because it worked for your second cousin on your father's side doesn't mean it's going to work for me.

The people who scare and upset me with their questions: 'Will you need surgery?' 'Will you ever work again?' 'Imagine how bad you're going to be when you are 60.' 'Will you need a wheelchair?' 'Did you know people with rheumatoid arthritis die younger?'

I'm very lucky to have two sons, but it's in my mom role that I am the biggest liar of all. My eldest son is autistic and anxiety is a huge issue for him, especially around medical issues and procedures. The smallest remark can set us back weeks or even months in the progress we have made with him.

If he saw me struggling with pain, he would instantly think that my death is imminent, that's just where his mind goes. So, if for example I've been driving for too long and pain is shooting through my knees, I fight back the tears and ensure that my sons don't see me suffering. Or if I drop a plate because the grip went in my hand, I make a joke about my butter fingers. In their eyes, mom and dad are invincible, so invincible is what I will pretend to be.

They know some of it, they know that the tablets I take are for the pains in my bones. They know that the injection I administer myself twice a week is also for my sore hands. But if my eldest asks about my day and I tell him I had a doctor's appointment, you see it; that flash of panic across his face. He asks what for and I talk it down to being a check-up, 'just making sure that mom is healthy'. That's all he can take right now.

No need to tell him that mom's painkillers have been doubled again in an effort to let her get some decent sleep, or that mom's anaemic again for some unknown reason and that's why she keeps feeling like she might fall over. Nope, say nothing, hide it. TMI as my kids would say.

Rheumatoid arthritis has taken a lot from me. In 2012, a redundancy payment gave me the start-up money I needed to set up a business doing something I loved with the added bonus of being able to do it from home. I developed a very successful, profitable business with a large and loyal client base. I was well known for my reputation of producing a quality product with excellent service. But the late hours, the administrative demands and constant deadlines damn near killed me. I was a one-woman show.

I worked so hard that I didn't stop to pay heed to how crappy I had started to feel physically. It wasn't until my GP sent me to A&E with suspected sepsis that I really woke up and realised that while my mind might have been functioning at 100%, my body sure as hell wasn't. Physically, I was falling apart.

It's one thing to walk away from a business venture that

just didn't work out, maybe you can take some solace in the fact that you gave it your best shot and took that plunge. But when your business is thriving and you're at the point of being able to expand and explore the gazillion other ideas you have spinning around your brain until BOOM… rheumatoid arthritis rears its ugly head and reminds you of its presence in your body.

Throw in some nerve damage, tendon damage and a helping of fibromyalgia too just to really seal the deal and it's goodbye to the business I gave my heart and soul to for six amazing years.

Eighteen months later and I am still calling it a blip, a bad patch, a stubborn flare. The question I really want to ask my rheumatologist 'Is this my life now? Is this my new norm?' But I still can't trust myself to get the words out in front of him without collapsing into a sobbing wreck. I'm scared that I already know the answer.

So, instead I scheme, I read and I plan on what I can do next. I am a person who needs to be busy, I love working. My next entrepreneurial venture is in the pipeline, tailor-made to fit around the demands of my disease. It might make me a liar, but rheumatoid arthritis will not define me.

Liam Gaule

From an early age, I was very active and was mad into sports; hurling (my favourite), Gaelic football, rowing, athletics (both on the track and cross country) and cycling.

I had a few injuries along the way, including badly torn ligaments in my ankle, and torn ligaments and tendons in my left knee when I was 20, but I carried on playing football with my club, Graiguecullen in Laois.

I was 26 when I married Úna; we'd three children, Maria, William and Keith, aged five, three and one. I had a good job working as a baker in Crotty's Bakery in Carlow and everything was going well; life was good.

In 1976, I was training for football every Tuesday and Thursday from early April with the odd match on a Sunday. When training, I walked the one-and-a-half miles to Fr Maher Park, Graiguecullen where we trained. While walking, I noticed that both of my feet were sore on the way over, but when I started training the soreness went. Then on the way home, the soreness would return.

I thought maybe I'm not as fit as I should be, but after a few weeks I went to my GP to see what the problem was. Dr Kelly thought I had gout, so he made an appointment for me in the Richmond Hospital in Dublin with Dr Counihan, who was an old colleague and both were in medical school together.

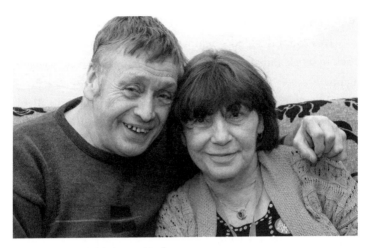

Liam Gaule with his late wife Úna

After numerous tests in the Richmond, Dr Counihan said 'Tell Joe he wasn't far out, but it's not gout you have, but rheumatoid arthritis.' The consequences of what he said did not hit me at the time, as I always thought that it was only older people who got arthritis, which I now know to be a myth.

I was put on a course of gold injections, but even so the RA spread to all my joints within a matter of a few weeks. With RA you can either lose or gain weight. Within one year, I went from being a fit 15st 7lbs to 10st 7lbs, the lowest weight I had been since I was 15 years old.

I often look back on photos from that era and I look a fright. Some of my friends even thought that I was dying.

After the gold injections, I was put on various anti-inflammatories and pain-killing medicines. I also tried natural remedies, including one which started with eating a pound of raw liver. At different times I cut out smoking and drinking. Over the years I put back on most of the weight I had lost.

In 1980 and 1981, I had the metatarsal bones in my feet

operated on, which gave me more comfort in walking.

In 1983, I decided – against the wishes of my GP – to go back to work and after a year I lost four stone and had to leave again.

That same year, Úna and I had our fourth child, Bríd, after a gap of eight years. When Úna told my mother that she was pregnant, my father overheard and said, 'I thought Liam had arthritis.' Úna replied, without missing a beat, 'Well, he hasn't got it down there!' That was funny, but it showed how people thought about the disease and the unusual ideas that sometimes exist. Two more daughters, Patricia and Nicole, arrived in 1985 and 1986.

In 1984, I had a few of what they called 'attacks' of arthritis, where all joints of the body were affected at the same time. I was referred to St James's Hospital in Dublin to be seen by a Mr Casey, the head rheumatologist.

The Arthritis Foundation organised a sponsored 100-mile walk in Boston in 1989, which I took part in – the only person on the walk with RA! While there, we paid a visit to the Brigham and Women's Hospital, which had great facilities for patients with arthritis.

That was a busy year. I went back to work in the bakery again – I hated being out of work – but had to give it up two years later, because I developed bursitis on my right elbow. My elbow would swell up, then it would be drained, but it would always return. Several tests followed, including a marrow test, but my elbow just got worse. Eventually, I was referred to an orthopaedic surgeon for a synovectomy (the removal of inflamed damaged tissues/bone from my elbow).

Sixteen weeks in hospital, surgery, physiotherapy – and slowly I regained a fair bit of use in my elbow, but lost a third of the flexibility.

In 1996, I was again admitted to St James's with very bad, consistent back pain and also to have the metatarsal in my right foot operated on again. I had some tests done and I remember the doctor coming to the ward, standing at my bed and saying 'Mr Gaule, we have good and bad news. We thought you might have cancer, but you haven't. The bad news is that you have spondylosis.'

Things were kind of normal from 1996-2004, although my left knee started to get really bad. It used to give way underneath me unexpectedly and many a time I almost fell.

Ultimately, I joined the waiting list for a knee replacement and after almost two-and-a-half years, I was given a choice of six hospitals. I chose Blackrock, simply because of the name.

I will always remember the day I went in, which was 2 December 2010, because it was the worst period of snow we had in years. I went up to Dublin on the train and I was fortunate to get a taxi from Heuston Station to the hospital, as nearly all the drivers had decided that it was too dangerous to drive.

I had the operation the next day. The surgeon, Dr Stefan Byrne, said to me he would love if I went to one of his lectures, so he could show people how a successful knee replacement should turn out. I think you could say he was pleased with his work.

Physio and rehab followed and on 23 December, I went home, just in time for Christmas.

It was a good move to go to Caritas for the rehab. The inclination is that if you decided to go home and do the exercises yourself, you would be inclined to say on some days, 'Ah sure, I'll take it easy today and do more tomorrow.' No chance of that in a rehab centre!

In 2013, I was diagnosed with COPD and at the same

time contracted TB. I gave up cigarettes as soon as I heard I had COPD.

Around this time, my rheumatologist changed my injections and I switched to a new biologic. Different medicines work differently for different people, so it is important not to be despondent if a certain medicine does not work as there are lots of treatments and sometimes it is by trial and error that you come by the right one.

When someone contracts arthritis, it is not the end of world. It just means that you have to adjust to a different lifestyle. RA can affect your mental state, so it is imperative to maintain a positive outlook.

I found that there are a few ways of dealing with RA. You can take the self-pity route and resign yourself to it or you can try and improve the situation by being positive and getting on with life. Just remember no matter how bad you are there is always someone worse off than you.

I remember in the first year I attended a clinic for my RA, I was feeling a bit down, thinking of all I was missing out on at work and sport, when I met a 45-year-old woman from Offaly, who was a farmer's wife and she told me her story. She said that she was working around the farm, milking cows and the like, when all of a sudden she got RA. Within a matter of a few weeks, she was in a wheelchair and her hands were so bad that she had to have a special gadget on her finger to hold a cigarette.

Talking to that woman made me realise that there were many people who were far worse off than me. There is help out there, from the likes of Arthritis Ireland, but the best help of all comes from your family and friends.

In that respect, I was very lucky as I had great support from my wife Úna (who sadly died nearly five years ago), my children, my grandchildren and my extended family and friends.

Arthritis can be hereditary and although none of my children got arthritis, one of my granddaughters, Ciara, got juvenile arthritis at two years of age. She is now 11 and seems be growing out of it as she gets older. Please God that will be the case.

For myself, my right knee and both hips have deteriorated and I am now waiting on an appointment to see an orthopaedic surgeon. I am also waiting for an appointment in the pain management clinic.

RA has been a part of my life for over 43 years and I have learned through time how to deal with it a lot better than I did at the beginning. The main thing I found was not to let it get you down and to try and have a positive outlook.

Robert Gawley

Before I start, can I just say I'm no writer or no big speech-maker? Nor do I talk much about my arthritis to ordinary folk or strangers; this is probably the first time I've really opened up about it and remembering back to those tough years.

My family are the only ones that know how much I suffered in those first three years. None more than my wife, who had to endure most of it. They say sometimes it's harder for the person looking on; even though I was the one living with this awful 24/7 pain. People close to you live the pain as well. My wife has been my rock through all this and I love her so much for it.

At 34, I was six years married, had two lovely twin boys, who were seven years old and was generally a very contented working guy. For about a week, I noticed I had a pain in my foot that was causing me discomfort and I was probably limping at the time. After about two or three weeks of pain, I was struggling when I lifted up my arm.

So, I took painkillers and got on with life, like anyone else. I was never one to go to doctors or anything. Although, in general, my health was very good, now I was noticing a few things about myself.

My pain seemed to be spreading to different parts of

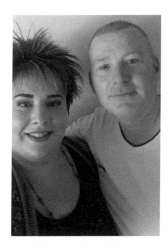

Robert Gawley with his wife, Emma

my body. At work, while I was moving around a lot, the pain didn't seem too bad. When I got home from work though, once I stopped moving, my whole body was aching; like the Tin Man in the Wizard of Oz when he didn't have oil in his joints. That was me, I just couldn't do anything.

Another thing I noticed when I got in from night shift, I was exhausted; in fact, I was constantly tired, I just wanted to be left alone to sleep all day. And, something I regret a lot, even now it still bugs me, I was becoming a pain to live with. I was on edge all the time; my wife couldn't talk to me without getting a short tempered remark back.

All my two boys wanted to do was go to the park and play football or games with their daddy, but I was just too tired and sore. Years later, I went for counselling, as I felt I let my wife and kids down. The RA robbed me of time with my kids; time I won't get back.

I've struggled with this for years and still do a bit. To be truthful, the pain and fatigue was taking over my life. I was changing as a person, my personality, my thoughts, the way I was looking at my life was all changing. Even now as

I'm writing this, I'm remembering back to how low I felt in myself as a person.

After about four months of being tired and in constant pain, I decided it was time to go to the doctor. The first visit didn't go well. I remember explaining my symptoms, but he didn't seem too concerned. He put me on an anti-inflammatory and the nurse took my bloods.

At the start, the anti-inflammatory worked, but after about a month it stopped having any real effect, but I continued to take it nonetheless.

By Christmas, I was really really suffering. Sitting was sore, getting up and down stairs was painful. Everything I did was such a chore because of the pain I was in. The straw that broke the camel's back came on Christmas Eve. For any parent, that's a night you enjoy with your kids, putting them to bed and telling them Santa will be there in the morning and watching their excited faces.

I tried. I really really tried my best, but it all got too much for me when I was in so much pain on the floor trying to put up a wrestling ring for my two sons.

I couldn't do it. I broke down on the floor crying. I'd had enough, a 35-year-old dad crying in pain and wondering why, why me, why not the guy next door or the person in the next street?

I felt like I was getting picked on by some higher force. I was so angry. I know it sounds silly, but this is the way I thought; I'm a good person, why has this happened to me?

My wife turned to me and said, 'That's it, we're both seeing the doctor after Christmas to find out what's going on.'

That visit to the doctors went much better, my wife was with me this time and after getting more blood results back, the doctor said, 'I think we need to refer you to a rheumatologist, the ESR levels in your blood are quite high.' I thought to myself, finally I'm being taken seriously, this isn't just all in my head.

The first rheumatology appointment was a bit underwhelming if I'm being honest. I had built myself up that the rheumatologist was going to give me an answer or a tablet that would help take this pain away.

Instead, I had to get more bloods done, get x-rays and an MRI.

A month later, the results were back. I'll never forget her words: 'Mr Gawley, you've got rheumatoid arthritis, now this is how we will go about treating you.'

Music to my ears, I'm gonna be pain-free; happy days, I thought. Not quite. There were side effects to this drug, which was a DMARD (disease-modifying anti-rheumatic drug). They seemed to go on and on... I had to watch what I eat, get regular bloods done, it could affect my liver, not drink. I had lots of questions.

It was a lot to take in on that first day. First of all, I was told I've got rheumatoid arthritis and there's no cure, but it can be managed by medication. But there are side effects. I know it sounds stupid, but I felt on one hand I'm pain free, which is fantastic, but on the other hand, there are certain things I can't do and eat in case it upsets my liver. Like just having a beer with friends, round at a barbecue. In my head, it's like this arthritis thing is actually ruling my life!

The rheumatologist was right about the side effects. I had to take six tablets every Tuesday, along with another drug. Although the drug worked for me and I was more or less pain-free, there was a massive downside. I just couldn't seem to stomach these tiny tablets; they made me ill and feeling nauseous all the time. I couldn't eat, even smelling food made feel sick.

I tried anti-sickness tablets, I was told cut the tablets back to four, I had a hospital phone number, where one of the rheumatology nurses would answer any of my concerns. I hated that drug and I know it works for a lot of people, but I just felt so depressed, so low in myself being sick, weak and tired all the time.

At one point, I said to my wife, 'You know what, love, I think I'd rather have the pain back, this is actually worse.' And I felt so selfish for saying that. Everyone was trying to do their best for me and I didn't want this medication anymore.

It was agreed at my next review with the rheumatologist that I would try a different DMARD. Unfortunately, this one didn't do much for me either, but it made me feel very spaced-out, like I was in a bubble or something. At one point, I felt like I was going to black-out, so needless to say, I was taken off this medication and went back on steroids.

At my next rheumatology appointment, we spoke about my symptoms, the drugs that weren't working and their side effects. Despite feeling very disheartened, the rheumatologist offered us hope by explaining that there were lots of other options, including biologics. Driving home, my wife and I were hoping and praying that I would qualify for one of the biologic drugs.

I remember the day when we received our answer like it was yesterday; waiting nervously to be called in by the rheumatologist. I don't know who was more nervous, me, or my wife – who had watched me go through every emotion, every injection, every appointment. It was a hard journey for her as well. Emma always told me, we'll get through this together. I honestly don't know what I would have done without her support; I owe her so much.

When we met with the rheumatologist, she handed me a

simple outline drawing of a person and asked me to mark the areas where I was experiencing pain.

Where wasn't I?

The shoulders, buttocks, hands, wrists, fingers, knees, jaw and neck were all duly marked on the poor unsuspecting cartoon man. A few more questions followed and the rheumatologist left the room. When she came back, she carried the news we'd be waiting to hear, I qualified for the biologic. I turned to my wife, who was actually crying, as the emotion took over.

I'm still on that drug four years on, injecting myself every fortnight. Although I still get flair-ups and pain now and again, that drug has given me my life back.

Rheumatoid arthritis has changed me. I'm not the same person I was before it happened. I've had counselling and at times suffer from depression, but it's also shown me life is precious and not to be taken for granted.

I've never talked openly about my arthritis before; I never really thought anyone would want to listen, but writing this and looking back, I'm saying to myself, there could be someone in a similar position to where I was.

All I can say is, you will get through it. It's hard, really hard at times, but don't do it on your own, talk to people and get as much information as you can. You will get there; I did.

Claire Geary

I suppose we all have our own story to tell and each is equally important, and it would be nice to think that we may all learn something new or helpful from each other's story.

For me arthritis is a cruel disease and one that for many years has had a negative impact on my life – but in other ways it has taught me to appreciate what I have… so here goes my story.

We got married in August 1997, and at 11.05pm on 5 April 2006 our gorgeous son Alex was born – albeit 10 days 'late' – 19 hours of labour ending in an emergency c-section; it was quite the dramatic entrance to this world.

Towards the middle of that April, I started to get stiff and found it hard to get out of bed in the mornings, then by late April, the stiffness had turned to discomfort in both ankles. I put it down to the fact that I am 5ft 4" and had carried a 9lb 10oz baby, so the end of the pregnancy was tough, particularly on my back, and then the birth was a bit dramatic. So, I just ignored it and muddled on. Like most new mums, I had a lot on my plate with my baby.

I turned 35 on 3 May and it was by this time that I could say the 'real' pain started. I found it very hard to walk in the mornings, so I booked to see my GP. I'm quite a tough cookie, so it takes a lot for me to visit my GP and she has known

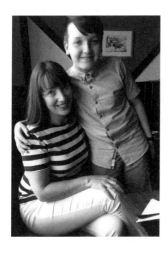

Claire Geary with her son Alex

me years. She took great care in listening to me and before I left her surgery that day, she had bloods sent off and told me honestly that she felt it was arthritis. BOOM! I did not see that coming.

For the next day or two, I suppose I thought 'why me', is arthritis not just for 'old' people? I remember seeing people with 'claw-like fingers' and worried this would happen to me. My GP called me within a week and said she was sorry, it was confirmed as rheumathoid arthritis and it was quite bad, so she was faxing a prescription to the pharmacy for painkillers and steroids and was arranging for me to see a consultant.

I got my head together with my little cocktail of drugs, and I though, right, RA let's be having you, and stupidly I thought this was as bad as it was going to get. I thought that as I was on medicines it would only improve, but I wasn't going to be that lucky.

My appointment for the consultant was within two weeks, so not much time to wait, but even in that time the pain was escalating and by now it was in both ankles, both knees, both shoulders, and from the soles of my feet to the tips of my toes. I was in and out to my GP taking more painkillers and the pain was so bad I was hunched over at the shoulders and I couldn't straighten my neck.

I felt so tired and upset that these precious months with my new baby were being taken away from me. My family were not living near enough to pop in and help, so I was really on my own until my husband came home from work.

I felt it was a blessing having my son, as it made me get up and move around, rather than just curling up in bed, feeling sorry for myself.

My first visit to the consultant was an eye-opener, he's a direct type of chap, no mollycoddling which actually suited me quite well. He showed me pictures, explained what was happening and why it was happening, my symptoms were quite severe and he explained it would take time to get me 'sorted', but he was confident we had caught it early and the outlook was good. He mentioned it would take a few months to get the right balance of the medicines, but it ended up taking almost a year.

I met a lovely rheumathology nurse who showed me how to do my injections (practice on an orange first; hah! that didn't work for me). I must have spent an hour my first day sitting at the kitchen table with the syringe trying to stick it into my leg.

So, the next few months are a bit of a blur, it seemed like GP … consultant … change meds … repeat.

By December there was a bit of an improvement, so I just focused on that and hoped for the best. I got out for more walks with the pram, started cooking (to be honest, at 35 years of age I learned to cook using the Annabel Karmel baby cookbook), but it was easy and quick and I wanted to reap the benefits of fresh home-cooked meals and I avoided processed/convenience foods as much as possible.

By March 2007, I started to think about the baby's first birthday, but around the same time I got a really bad flare-up and nothing was working, so I had to go to hospital and have intravenous infusions. By mid-April, I was feeling much better, but taking so many tablets, my husband used to say that if you shook me, I'd rattle like a smarty box, as I also took medicine for my thyroid.

I look back now and wince at the memory of trying to 'pop' those tiny little baby fasteners on the baby grows – omg, there were like torture instruments. It could take me 15 minutes just to change a nappy and get him dressed again. Tiny buttons and buttonholes broke my heart.

But my son was great, it's like he knew something was up. He never struggled when I changed him, from a young age he'd grip me around my neck and hold on as I'd lift him. At six months he was holding his own bottle, from day one he only woke once or twice at night and when he was about 16 weeks old, he started sleeping through the night. It was such a help to me having such an easy baby.

One of the toughest times was when the RA started to affect my eyes. This meant a number of trips to hospital to sort out, copious amounts of eyedrops and eventually it eased off. But they were so dry, any light at all hurt them, so even indoors I had to wear sunglasses, which kind of made me stand out at work – people probably thought I was trying to start a new trend!

My own struggles were very real and, unfortunately, I had an employer at the time who was appalling in how they treated me. I had to give up work and thought I'd never work again, but I was wrong and things did improve. By the time my son was three years old, I was doing well, so I went to work part-time at a local pharmacy and stayed there for five years, until the RA acted up and my poor feet just could not handle standing any more.

Three or four hours into the day, every step I took was agony. I spent a fortune on the best of shoes to comfort my feet. Comfortable they may have been, but they were in no way stylish and I just tried to hide them behind the counter!

Eventually it got too much and it was very sad to leave a job that I loved. Chatting with my GP, we felt that maybe going back to a desk job might suit me better, so I sent my CV to a highly regarded firm that was just 15 minutes' drive from my home. I was a bit nervous as they are involved in the health industry and had quite an extensive medical form to fill in. But I took a chance and filled it in honestly, gave them permission to speak with both my GP and consultant, and they offered me a full-time role with them. I was thrilled, but not sure how I'd fare out doing five full days but I said I'd give it a go.

So, five-and-a-half years later and I am still with the same company and still working full-time, a few flare-ups along the way, but thankfully nothing too serious. The initial biologic stopped working for me, so I am now on a different one and kept on a DMARD (disease-modifying anti-rheumatic drug). I am delighted that for a number of years now, I have had very little need to take anti-inflammatory tablets. I am also in a very lucky position to be able to work from home, with an employer that offers great support.

I will be honest and say that for a while, I thought this was the worst thing that could have happened to me, but it's not, it's just bad luck.

I like to walk, get out for small runs, I do a lot of needlework and find this is really great for my fingers. RA has not stopped me from doing anything – maybe I have had to adapt some areas of life, but I have not given up anything.

I have a very positive outlook on life, I look after myself, keep fit and eat very healthily and all these combined definitely make me feel better. I wake up every morning, pop in my eye drops and do my stretches even before I get out of the bed.

If someone was to ask me today what is the hardest part of my RA to deal with, I would say without a doubt it's the fatigue. While I can work a full day, I am limited, or in some cases, not able to do anything in the evening. Or if I tackle housework, I might get an hour's work done, but then have to rest.

I've learned that when I am really tired, I just have to have a nap – I literally cannot keep my eyes open. I have been known to start falling asleep at the table eating dinner. Long family days are very tough too, like a communion or wedding, I might need one or two power naps just to get me through the day. Late nights are a thing of the past, if I make it to 11.30 on a night out I'm doing well.

Early diagnosis is key, so if you have a strange ache or pain, please see your GP. Hopefully it will be nothing serious, but if it is RA, the earlier you are diagnosed and get help the better. I was lucky to get an early diagnosis and thankfully was able to pay to see a private consultant; I know not everyone can, but having this consultant made a huge difference to me.

Thank you for reading my story, maybe it will give hope to someone newly diagnosed, that while there will be some tough days, hopefully it will get better for you like it did for me.

Siobhán Grehan

Crystal clear water and beams of illuminating sunlight reflecting on iridescent fish above a floor of golden dust – I had done it! Fifty years young and I was scuba diving off the coast of Cyprus, where even the seawater is warm.

Just me, the bubbling sound of my air tank and freedom... and Scuba Steve following close behind with a camera. My personal guard and guide as I ticked off my bucket list, made all the more impressive considering my secret claustrophobia.

The arrival of my fiftieth birthday had focused my mind on the singularity of life, its ever increasing speed and the unpredictable route it takes. Like so many women of my age and position; a mother, wife, daughter and career woman – all rolled into one, my dreams, goals and ambitions had turned into a burning desire for my children's happiness and success, in whatever form that might take.

Today it seems they have eternal youth, a travel lust and a millennial attitude that their parents had it so much easier; maybe they are right, but who's to say.

Soon after my third child/adult finally passed their driving test, I started to think surely my work here is done and it is time to be my own priority. I consider myself to be an optimistic realist.

I like to solve problems, I never bury my head in the

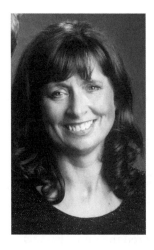

Siobhán Grehan

sand and a little over 30 years ago, I was lucky enough to marry a man with a very similar disposition, quite the recipe for success. At this point, you are probably thinking that this is supposed to be my rheumatoid arthritis story and yet I haven't mentioned it, but there are so many things in my life both before and after RA, and it is simply an unwelcome diagnosis that arrived 22 years ago.

It was 1997 when I got diagnosed; I had three very young children, was still changing nappies and carrying a toddler up to bed. We had just moved to a house that quickly became a building site, life was happy and chaotic. Somewhere in the process I developed a red, hot, swollen and most of all, very painful, right hand and wrist. There followed a long, drawn out saga of doctors, blood tests, x-rays, physiotherapy and drugs – with little improvement.

Eventually I moved up a level and a consultant ordered an MRI, which gave a choice of two diagnoses, one of which was RA, but in the absence of many of the typical symptoms of RA we went with RSD (no need to explain, because apart from a tendon injected with steroids and intensive painful physio this diagnosis didn't stick). It took a couple more weeks of pain before things finally pointed us to the correct diagnosis – RA.

I was 32 and all I could think of was an elderly lady on the first medical ward I worked on in Dr Steevens' Hospital, as a student nurse barely 18 years of age. I remembered the lady so well; she was admitted in a RA flare-up, every joint in her body was affected, she couldn't straighten her limbs and her hands were curled, deformed and useless. It stuck with me how appreciative she was of every little thing we did for her and that she never complained.

It was unthinkable that I now shared the same diagnosis. There followed a thankfully brief period of utter panic, my mind raced in every direction trying to run every possible scenario for every future situation, giving new meaning to the expression 'analysis paralysis'.

Thankfully, the problem solving, realistic, optimistic part of me took control. I finally had a correct diagnosis and a battle plan; I would take the medication, on this occasion a DMARD (disease-modifying anti-rheumatic drug), anti-inflammatories and painkillers and I would be a willing team player with my team of occupational therapists and physiotherapists. The resting splints and working supports they so expertly made were my friends, even if my children named one splint 'The Claw'.

Years passed, the drugs worked and RA was held at bay, ever hovering in the wings. My plan had been to fully embrace all aspects of my treatment and my goal was to be symptom-free with no long-term joint damage.

I settled for what I got, which was less than what I wanted. The inflammation in my right hand had lasted for so long before the disease became inactive, I now had severe arthropathy (there is one to google), permanent bone change and reduced joint function, so time to adapt. After a number of years with good blood results and no joint inflammation, I was even released from taking medication.

Years passed, my family grew up and life raced on until gradually getting up in the morning got uncharacteristically slower and one knee was painful and swollen, but this time I recognised my old adversary and when the pain started in both hands and feet it was no surprise to me when the blood test confirmed it was back. My weapon of choice this time was a different DMARD; the side effects made for some sobering reading; thankfully, I wasn't planning any more pregnancies and I wasn't bothered by the regular blood tests, even the alcohol consumption restrictions were fine, as long as it worked.

It did, quickly starting on a low dose and building up it worked in weeks. It's been years now and though the dose is lower, I still reluctantly take my weekly dose knowing the unpleasant after effects for the day, but it is worth it.

This second battle extended the damage to my right wrist to affect my thumb joint too and again time to adapt.

If my story is to be truthful, I have to mention fatigue! Although I would rather not, it is the symptom I find hardest to acknowledge and probably the least understood. There is no blood test, x-ray or scan that will confirm its existence, but for those who have experienced it, they will understand its effect on physical, emotional, social and cognitive function.

When someone says they are tired, even exhausted, it is my experience that the most common response is 'So am I.' There is a sign I see regularly on a major road near where I live that reads 'Tiredness Kills'. The truth is not that tiredness kills, but it is the way it affects our ability to drive that can be fatal. We have all seen the driving ads, pull in, take a nap, have a coffee and then off you go again – problem solved.

Unfortunately, it does not work that way with RA and personally I am not a fan of naps, I would rather go to bed early. So, for what it's worth, my coping strategy: early to bed (when needed), exercise within your limits (that means walking for me), healthy diet and then just live your life.

RA is just part of my story, we are acquaintances now and for life. I know my limits, I don't always stay within them, but there are things I will simply never do because of them, and that is absolutely fine.

So, I may not shake your hand firmly anymore, but I will travel, meet people and have adventures. Just living within my limits, most of the time!

Annette Haran

When I was diagnosed with rheumatoid arthritis at the age of 46, I was shocked and upset. You see, I knew what it was, my aunt and her daughter (my first cousin) had it, in very severe forms. Both had been in wheelchairs and both had died in their fifties by the time I was diagnosed. I had a lot of pain and stiffness especially in my hands. The future looked very bleak.

The rheumatologist said, 'There is no cure for it, but it won't kill you', which I didn't believe at the time. While there are lots of different drugs for treating RA, they each have their own side effects. I ended up in hospital for a week with a severe reaction to one of the meds.

Somehow, I just keep pushing through the good days, meaning I have a bit of energy and very little pain; on bad days it's like my whole body is in pain, I've no energy and am very emotional. I try very hard not to give in to this, so I am probably very cranky on those days.

I've experienced lots of side effects over the years, ranging from nausea, severe headaches, very bad mouth ulcers, constant ear infections, diverticulitis (which I was hospitalised with on several occasions), high blood pressure and cholesterol. I had a severe reaction to one drug which left me looking like I had no skin I was so red, my head was all swollen and my ears were like cabbage leaves, the very big green ones. I was in the high dependency unit for a few days.

After that harrowing experience, I was put on monthly infusions. I had a long drive on my own to the hospital and I constantly had problems with my veins. I did this for around seven years. Thankfully, I was started on a new drug about two years ago and it is working well for me.

For me, RA is pain in my joints, it's soreness and it's heat that I cannot cool, it's stiffness and fatigue. At times, it is depressing, especially when something is planned with family or friends when it strikes. It's random, my feet and hands today; yesterday it was my hips, the back of my neck and my breast bone.

I look fine, although my weight has almost doubled in the 15 years since I was diagnosed, largely due to the meds. I also have an underactive thyroid, which slows the metabolism. That's the thing, you rarely have just one autoimmune disease.

I don't work outside the home now and this is probably the thing I grieve most. It has become hard to do simple tasks. I worked for a fashion designer many years ago, and any kind of crafting is my passion. I always loved to do my own interior design, including updating furniture or painting the house. Unfortunately, that has almost disappeared from my life.

Cutting vegetables or opening bottles and jars are sometimes impossible for me. Having to stand for even a short time is crippling, queuing is a no-no really, unless it is a very short queue. When I do housework, I get really tired, my hands, feet and ankles get very hot and swollen. Flat shoes do not suit me at all, I can't walk very long without getting pain in my feet, but with flats I have no chance.

This is something many people can't understand, because for me, there is no such thing as comfortable shoes with RA.

If I am going somewhere, I have to think about where I will park, how far I will have to walk, will the ground be flat, are there steps to climb, if so how many. It's terrible sometimes to walk across a big car park in pain and when you get near the entrance, there are several empty parking spaces that you can't park in. I don't have a parking permit; I'm not entitled to one apparently. If you can walk, pain doesn't count it seems.

Sometimes, crossing the road I can be slow and because I don't look like the typical little old lady, I get abuse and people blowing the horn at me. I can get infections very easily because my immune system is compromised, and so bring hand sanitizer with me all the time.

When I have very bad days, I stay away from people, because most don't understand what's going on. Some things people say really annoy me – and everyone with RA gets these. 'Oh, but you *look* great', as if there couldn't be anything wrong because I got dressed-up or put on some make-up. 'My grandmother had that and she lived to be 95' and, of course, the old chestnut, 'Sure, you're too young to have arthritis.'

One of the challenges of rheumatoid arthritis is the word 'arthritis'. Most people think of it only as an old person's disease, without realising that it can affect anyone – of any age, and that it is more than just joint pain. Anything that could inform people or increase understanding of the challenges of living with the condition would be welcome.

I am blessed to have fantastic grandchildren and I would like to be able to do more with them. I exercise as much as I can, I do yoga, use the hydrotherapy pool regularly and from time to time go to the gym.

RA is an expensive disease, especially when you don't have a medical card, between medicines, blood tests, consultant appointments, visits to the GP…

It can all sound very doom and gloom, but it's not really. I have gotten used to it to a large degree and can manage it pretty well. Little gadgets that make chores easier to do help, support groups like Arthritis Ireland and others on Facebook are very supportive and I have learned a lot from them. I have an amazing medical team, for which I am grateful, and while it might sound strange, but I am also grateful for the drug companies who do all the research and develop new treatments.

I'm not worried about going into a wheelchair anymore. I still look fine.

Sally Harron

My story begins in 1979 when I was aged 21. I was married three years at this time and I was a telephonist in the local phone exchange.

It began with pains in my fingers and wrists, and progressed to my elbows and shoulders. When I went to my GP, he said it was probably tendonitis, resulting from my work at the telephone exchange with my hands. The pains continued and then I noticed that my toes were getting sore too, and I thought this could not be related to my telephonist work.

I saw some more doctors, who told me it might be viral, maybe stress, maybe overworking the arms, maybe I should stop walking to and from work.

Any time I went to the GP, he would give me a pain-killing injection into whatever joint was troubling me, including my toes; the pain of these injections was horrendous. And, so I continued with hot packs, ice packs, wrist bandages, anything that would give me ease, in fact, for six years.

One day, my older sister told me she would take me to another town where she worked and made an appointment for me with her GP and I told him the whole story. Now 28, he examined me, took some blood tests and told me to return in a week, which I did.

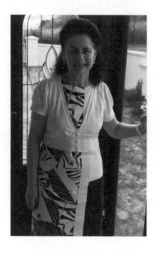

Sally Harron

'I have got to the bottom of the problem you are having with joint pain,' he said. 'Oh, that's great,' was my immediate reply, hugely relieved because I felt everyone was questioning my sanity at this stage.

'Well, it's not great really, because you have rheumatoid arthritis, which is a very debilitating disease and can often leave a person crippled or even wheelchair-bound.'

Scarcely acknowledging what the doctor had just said, I replied I was relieved to get the diagnosis and would have to cope, whichever way I could. Leaving the surgery with a printout of the blood results, I took these to my local GP, who said he had already tested me for that and nothing showed up.

On another visit to the doctor sometime later, another GP was standing-in and he suggested that I see a rheumatologist. I'd never heard the word. He referred me to Dr Raman, consultant rheumatologist at Our Lady's Hospital in Manorhamilton, Co. Leitrim, a two-hour drive from my home.

On that first appointment, he said I need to admit you to the hospital for at least two weeks to see if we can get your ESR down and get your disease managed. I hadn't a clue what he was talking about. I was admitted to the ward and stayed there for three weeks – getting injections, drips, physiotherapy and medication – and left feeling much better.

I continued to attend Dr Raman at an outpatient clinic in Letterkenny, and whenever I had flare-ups, was admitted to the hospital in Co. Leitrim, as there was no rheumatology ward in Letterkenny General Hospital.

While I told my husband and family about my RA, I instructed them not to tell anyone else that I had arthritis, as I felt it was an old person's disease. The only person I knew with pains was my granny; I felt ashamed and embarrassed.

One day, in the hospital I picked up a magazine with Arthritis Ireland on the cover, and in an article found the names of two people in their office: Ruth Findlater and Brian Crotty.

I phoned Ruth and asked if there were any arthritis support groups in Donegal; there weren't, but she asked if I might be interested in starting one. I was, because I had learned of another girl with arthritis who was the same age as me, and I wanted to get to know more people with the condition, not just old people!

Marian Gordon and I duly met with Ruth, and we set-up a branch in Donegal. That was 1987 and Marian and I are great friends to this day. Loads of younger people turned up at meetings and it was fantastic.

I went through the usual anti-inflammatories, ACTH drips, disease-modifying drugs (DMARDs) and gold injections. I had a severe reaction to the gold injections and had to stop them. Then I developed a rash every now and then, and had other problems with my health.

One day, my rheumatologist told me that I also had

systemic lupus erythematosus (SLE) or simply lupus. I told him I wasn't bothered about names and labels; I was only interested in keeping mobile and keeping going as long as I could unaided.

I continued to attend Manorhamilton hospital and through the Donegal branch of Arthritis Ireland, we were instrumental in fundraising for a hydrotherapy pool there, which is a great benefit to people with arthritis, and indeed MS and stroke patients too.

I was chairperson of the Donegal branch for 25 years and retired from the position by making a presentation for arthritis research at a function in Letterkenny. I enjoyed my time with the branch and can honestly say that the day I made that phone call to Ruth Findlater was the best day of my life, as I was in the depths of despair thinking I was the only young person with this disease.

I am very grateful to my husband, Dinny, who stood by me all the years and supported and cared for me in every way, and was never embarrassed to go out with me while I was on crutches or wearing different hand and arm bandages. He took me to all the clinics when I couldn't drive or change gears, and summer or winter came to see me in hospital. Without his love and support, my life would have been very difficult and very different.

I have continued through all of the years and worked in my local Clonleigh Coop for the past 35 years, where my employer was very understanding of my illness and always allowed me any time off that I needed to attend hospital or appointments or indeed time off to rest up at home. Without this support, I would not have been able to lead a normal life, and for that I am grateful to Jim Patterson and Gareth Patterson.

I am now 63 years old and feel that the pain today is not nearly as bad as it was when I was 22 – or maybe you just get used to a certain amount of discomfort every day; in any case it is now bearable.

My painful regrets about having RA and SLE is that they robbed me of a family and of the best years of my life; when everyone else was out enjoying themselves, I was laid up at home often crying with pain. Such is life, and you have to take what is dealt out to you.

In another way, it has made me, I hope, a better person and I really feel for and sympathise with people who have a disability, and maybe if I never had RA maybe I would not be that person.

That's my RA story.

Ann Marie Healy

The west of Ireland rural village where I was born is still my home. Being the fifth child born into a family of 16 children, my childhood was a happy one.

I was five years of age when my family first took me to the local doctor. My parents were traumatised to hear I had rheumatic fever, as other family members already had the disease.

Hospital stays and pain medication soon became my life. Through my early school years, a lack of energy and dealing with pain made those years very difficult. By age 10, there were already concerns, as my neck was stiff and my finger joints were showing signs of juvenile rheumatoid arthritis.

By the time I was in my teenage years, damage was already being caused to my joints because of the arthritis. I continued my schooling, completing my leaving cert in an all-Irish school, Coláiste Chomáin, Rossport, Co. Mayo. By this time, it was necessary for me to have corrective surgery on my right hand, as I was having difficulty writing and carrying out everyday tasks. This was the start of many surgeries.

Despite this, I got on with life and have looked for opportunities to further my education. With a keen interest in and love of country music, it's given me opportunities to get out and socialise.

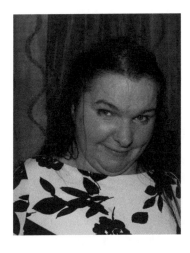

Ann Marie Healy

Over the years, I have had about 40 surgeries, including having knuckle, hips, knees, shoulders and elbow replacements, as well as neck and foot surgeries.

Now a wheelchair user, the Erris branch of the Wheelchair Association was a great help and support to me. Over the years, in turn, I represented them on their regional and national executive councils, as well as on the local committee.

I joined the Centre for Independent Living, Mayo and they provided me with a personal assistant, who greatly enhanced the quality of my life. Independent living is multifaceted in its approach and includes supports for my personal needs and mobility. For instance, I couldn't drive myself because of the arthritis in my fingers and elbow joints, so I had to rely on my personal assistant and family to bring me wherever I wanted to go. Without this support, I would not have been able to live my life to the fullest. I'm glad to say that I've also been able to give back, and so I worked with the centre as a leader coordinator, which I really enjoyed.

I also joined the Mayo branch of Arthritis Ireland and

am very involved with them across a wide range of activities – including lobbying for the appointment of a full-time rheumatologist in Mayo General Hospital, so that people with arthritis in the county don't have to travel to Dublin or Galway for treatment. Arthritis Ireland have also been a great support to me.

Being from a big family has its benefits. If any of my family knew that I needed assistance, they were always there to support me in achieving my goals, including pursuing several courses and achieving my dream of going to the Institute of Technology in Sligo where I studied social studies. Graduating with a diploma in social studies was a real highlight.

Throughout the years I kept diaries; it was a comfort to be able to put my feelings on paper. The idea of turning my diaries into a book came about later. Even though I had all this information in handwritten diaries, I had to think about what I would share with the public and rewriting those memories brought me back again and made me realise how difficult some of the periods in my life had been.

Dealing with a disability and fighting my corner for supports so that I could live an independent life has also been a feat at times. I have tried to keep positive, while my friends and the people I have met through my life have uplifted me and given me courage. Despite living with this ravaging disease and having to spend a lot of my life on metal wheels, I am a happy person.

Above all, I believe in moving forward all the time. It is very important for me to be active, as it distracts me from my pain.

One of the things which helped a lot was a self-management course, 'Living well with arthritis' which I completed in 2008. This greatly enhanced the quality of my life and helped me learn how to stay mentally and physically healthy. I have to work harder at this than most, because I don't cook and depend on support to put together healthy meals.

So, whether it's keeping sugary and fatty foods and salt to a minimum; eating fruit, vegetables, pasta and white meat; keeping physically active; getting regular physiotherapy or hydrotherapy – these all contribute to me living a healthy life.

To stay mentally active, I need to have goals, be around positive people, keep active and 'out there', participating in whatever's going on in the community, and being fulfilled in my life.

To this end, I have been busy with my book, I present a weekly programme on my local community radio station, I'm on the Erris Community Health Forum, and have undertaken a wide variety of courses from computing to healthcare support and nursing studies. It's a full and busy life.

One of the highlights of my life was being awarded Erris Person of the Year in 2008, which was a great confidence builder and it encouraged me to reach out to help others.

At 50, I feel I live a very full life. Even though I cannot see a cure for rheumatoid arthritis in my lifetime, I am positive that I can continue to live a full life and have confidence in a health system that is managing to control my pain.

If I had a million euros to spend, I would not want to change my life.

Maeve Horgan-Perle

I wish rheumatoid arthritis had a different name.

Y'see, so many people think they know what it is, and think they have experience with it; a few creaks, being a bit stiff as you get up off a chair, a few oul' aches and pains, ah sure 'tis only natural at our age...

The older I get, the harder it is to patiently keep the polite smile rigidly on my face when I hear offhand remarks like 'Me too! I have arthritis in my shoulder. Have you tried Epsom salts? Lovely hot bath'll fix you right up!' People mean well. They want you to feel better and so they're only dyin' to jump in and solve the problem. Only, y'see, they can't. It's just not that easy.

Let's start with what it's not. RA's not just a few aches and pains. Sit with that for a while and chew on it a few times.

It's not something two pills or taking a bath will ever solve. Nor will the new panacea of hope – CBD oil – cure it. Nope. Believe me I've tried!

It's a progressive disease that can affect the heart, the lungs, the eyes, your energy, cachexia (muscle-wasting), your ability to fight infections, and yes, the bones and joints. The joints all over your body – from the feet, to the knees, to the wrists, the fingers, your jaw, your neck... Ever break a bone? Well, imagine feeling like you had 17 of those pains in your

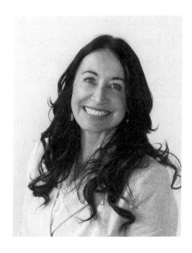

Maeve Horgan-Perle

body. Yep. it's way more serious than natural aging.

And, in much the same way that cancer has stages, so too does RA. Mild is relatively easy to manage with medication and any necessary lifestyle changes. Moderate will require some of the more serious medications and patience – expect some trial and error with a touch of two steps forward and one step back. And then there's severe RA. This is where your joints get so painful and so inflamed that you can't move them. Imagine both hands and feet not being able to bend?

Such was my experience in 2013; I went from being a fit, 45-year-old outdoors enthusiast, to not being able to dress myself.

The reason for someone developing RA has proved to be a mystery to doctors and scientists alike. Not too sure there's one reason. From my research, it's something that may have lain dormant in my genes, perhaps activated by trauma and/ or certain bacterial infections, compounded (or kept at bay) by lifestyle choices and nutrition, and maybe alleviated and exacerbated by hormonal changes. Probably a mishmash of all of the above.

When the diagnosis is first handed to you and you do some research, you get scared. My hands weren't moving and the internet told me that 50% of people with RA will give up work within five years, and then… muscle wasting, heart inflammation, the list went on.

Time to PANIC!!! And then comes the avalanche of confusing, guilty thoughts – trying to understand what on earth you've done to deserve this. I was a newly trained yoga teacher who guzzled green smoothies daily, who didn't smoke and who only drank at happy occasions, so y'know, what the whaaat…?

And then you read statistics that 70% of people with RA had childhood trauma, so you put your best Sherlock hat on, trying to unearth family secrets (probably imagined or otherwise), not to mention the futile hours of contemplation – the 'why me/poor me' questions.

At the very least, be prepared to cry. The complete and utter lack of understanding from well-meaning friends and family will hurt you. Know that now. Their lack of knowledge of what challenges you are facing will often seem insensitive and uncaring. Don't get me wrong – I have people. Lovely people. However, the 'Ah sure, you'll be grand' doesn't help. Not one feckin' bit!

Not when you are struggling to figure out how to put a bra on in the morning, not when you could get let go from your job because of sick days taken. Not when you are afraid of disability. Not when you are dealing with sick kids when you yourself are in pain. Not when you wonder if your partner will stay with the person you are becoming (as opposed to the vibrant, energetic being you were just a few years ago). Not when you lie awake at night, alone with the burden of trying to make your finances work if you go part-time….

Indeed, the pain and the worry associated with this disease can cause sleeplessness, which itself unearths a whole can of worms to deal with. I heartily suggest joining a rheumatoid arthritis support group where you can safely discuss your challenges, connecting with people offering solutions having been there themselves. Just be careful not to be overwhelmed by all of the challenges you hear about. It's unlikely you'll get all of them, I promise!

It takes a team of doctors to kick this disease into remission, so get thee to a rheumatologist, but talk with a naturopath doctor too. Try acupuncture, try an osteopath, a nutritionist – heck, try everything.

If I sound like an over-privileged git as I say this, forgive me. I know all of these cost money; however, trying all of these has been worth it in the end as I manage my disease. Yes, a diet full of unprocessed foods, foods low in sugar and an awful lot of green stuff will help, but it isn't enough. Hell, I've been friends with quinoa, on first name terms with spinach and have massaged kale with the best of 'em for years.

For sure, to reduce inflammation, good nutrition is a must. But alas, a healthy lifestyle isn't enough for severe RA. So, take the drugs, they'll keep your joints mobile and will hinder the progress of the disease. And do the hippy-gumbo stuff; nutrition, meditation (or prayer), gentle exercise, stress reduction techniques (sorry lads, wine doesn't count). Take a 360° approach and hit it with everything you've got at your disposal.

Speaking of drugs and steroids though, you can't afford to be flippant about what you are putting in your body. Addiction to painkillers and reliance on sleep medication is something you have to constantly monitor. Get in the habit of asking yourself if you have exhausted every single other option? Speaking of addiction, let's be honest. You'll probably be addicted to your own misery at the beginning too. At some stage, as the drugs begin to work, you get a reprieve and you'll realise you don't have the monopoly on misery. This will probably be a welcome relief to all.

Be aware that there can be some dubious physical side effects of the medication. Anal leakage, leprosy and erections lasting more than four hours, anyone? Ok, I may have made those up, but ya get my drift.

Seriously though. Try one drug at a time and journal how you are feeling so you can identify patterns when they happen. I felt lured, seduced. Attracted to the idea of floating down the river one evening having started a DMARD (a small dose of chemotherapy drugs – the first drug most doctors have you try). I wasn't depressed; it just changed my brain.

Poof! It happened just like that. I spoke up. I stopped the drug and it will never be used in my treatment again as the risk of suicide is real. So just be aware of any mood or physical changes. On the bright side, it catapulted me into studying positive psychology, the science of happiness and suicide prevention. So, there's that.

Friends, unless you are a rheumatologist with a bajillion years of medical experience and training, or a naturopath doctor or a GP, your job is to listen, to be compassionate. It certainly isn't to offer advice because you read some quack's opinion on the interwebs, or your neighbour's cousin told you. Yea, maybe your granny did have some nobbly fingers and cured what ailed her just by quitting gin. And yea, maybe your dodgy great-uncle with the Elvis toupee had RA and was still down the pub every evening. But, redirecting the conversation to some distant unknown is not what a person with RA needs.

They were hoping for a compassionate ear. In Irish there's a great saying – éist do bhéal – listen with your mouth (in other words, shut yours!). Don't make it about you. Sure, it may have hurt when you pulled a muscle in yoga, however our pain is not just in one place and is mental and physical and, more importantly, chronic (on-going).

Instead, ask what you can do to help. Doing odd jobs – anything from mowing the lawn, to dropping off a casserole or bringing your friend to the movies. Making a list of Netflix or Amazon binge-worthy series is a lovely thing to do when somebody is in a flare-up. Go over to their house to make yourself a cuppa tea and, sure while you're at it, make them one too. Organise walks or outings that they can do physically, showing patience and understanding. Send someone a care package (my fav's a box with paracetamol, Tayto and Irish Cadburys, thanks very much).

In short, it's not up to you to fix the problem; but as a loved one, sharing some of its burden will likely catapult you to saintly status.

When family want to bring their cutie-pie mucus monsters over to your house, learn to be firm and assertive if you don't want the kids (or sick adults) to come. People don't understand that your immune system (compromised by the disease and immune suppressant drugs) may not be able to fight this. And be OK with your friends being frustrated if you say no!

There are days when you are an invalid, and then there are days when you could put a Riverdance member to shame. You'll just have to get comfortable with being an intermittent moaning Mary for the next 30 odd years who needs to stay in bed every now and again.

As either a caregiver, family member, or a friend you

need to understand that your life may also change because we will not always be available to do the long-haul trips, weekend concerts, the midweek cheeky drinks at the local dive bar... Expecting somebody to bounce back because they've been sick for a while now, just isn't reasonable, we might be sick for two days or for six months. There is no logic to this disease – there are great days and not so great days. Of course, on your good days, make sure to return those favours and the kindnesses that have been shown to you.

Letting go of what you expected your life to be and embracing what is, is key to your happiness. Let go and let God (Buddha, Allah, Bono, Ganesh... whatever works for you).

Oh yea, Jeepers. I forget the fun part... not. It's esspennnnnsive. The price of the MRIs, the x-rays, the physical therapy, the specialists visits, the medications.

RA's not for the faint of heart. Lads, I could go on... indeed, the only way to deal with this is to have a gratitude practice about what IS good in your life... (and maybe to shell out an indecent sum of money on health insurance).

So, are there anything good things about RA? Well, my family and I are definitely eating healthier. I took up meditation and have all sorts of tricks for stress reduction that I have passed on to my family. I am significantly humbled by what I cannot do and this has led to me to be much more compassionate, patient and kind towards others. I know who my real friends are...

Recently, I put on my big-girl panties and studied positive psychology and wellness as I navigated living with this autoimmune disease. So, silver linings. Just be patient. Have hope. There are fun days ahead and always be grateful because it could be so, so much worse... Really.

Bernadette Kane

In November 2014 I had a procedure on my right hand to relieve carpal tunnel syndrome. Within two weeks, I was unable to lift my arms and had great difficulty putting on my coat or even combing my hair. My GP prescribed medication to relieve my symptoms, but it didn't work and I got progressively worse.

Early in the new year, I asked to be referred to a rheumatologist, had lots of tests done and was greatly relieved when I was diagnosed with RA. I felt I had a chance of getting to grips with my condition.

A supportive physiotherapist and numerous physiotherapy treatments helped greatly and I especially loved the 'hot wax' treatment on my hands and feet!

During the first year, my daily routine was to struggle out of bed, have a HOT shower (bliss!) and get dressed – which took about an hour struggling – total exhaustion! Breakfast – then to sofa – flick on TV – SLEEP – lunch – another struggle – and afternoon TV, but I made myself get up during the ads and walk around, then back on the sofa again! Dinner and nighttime TV was the same routine as lunch and the struggle to get ready for bed.

I made an effort to go for lunch once a week with a friend and I made sure I put on make-up whenever I went out and

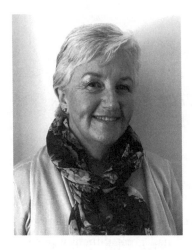

Bernadette Kane

had my hair cut short so I could manage it better

About a year later when I started to feel slightly better, I joined the local Arthritis Ireland group and did a self-management course, which was very good and extremely helpful, and I would recommend it.

I have always been an active, very busy person and found this 'new me' very strange and I was determined to get back to who I was before RA. Sometimes family celebrations afford those opportunities, so, in 2017, one of my daughters got married and I was thrilled to be able to join in the dancing at her wedding.

I'm now five years with the condition and must admit it has been a huge learning curve and I've gained an appreciation of what one can endure and overcome.

I'm back walking, sewing and doing art again. I've changed my diet and I'm a great believer in apple cider vinegar to help kick start my day. Diet plays a huge part in keeping symptoms at bay and I have to curb my sweet tooth at times – I'm winning, I think!

There are still bad days, but I'm now listening to my

body and find that when fatigue takes hold, I sit down, wrap up in a little fleece blanket, breathe in for five, hold for four and breath out for three a few times (I might even have 40 winks).

Afterwards I feel I can face life again and the light at the end of the tunnel is *not* the train coming at me, but the opening and the way forward!

Breda Kane

It's difficult to pinpoint when the symptoms started exactly. Looking back there were a few indications throughout the summer, but nothing that would have told me what was to come.

It was mid-October when I noticed that after work, I would find it difficult to climb the stairs to get to my apartment and that it was hard to press the off or volume buttons on the side of my phone. I'm a nurse, who works 13-hour shifts, so originally, I just put it down to being tired at the end of the day. I continued to get slightly worse, but I kept dismissing it as nothing, hoping that the symptoms would just go away, while promising my boyfriend that I'd go to the GP soon.

This continued until a Monday morning in November, I went to see my sister and nephew, who was nine months at the time. I was holding him for only five minutes before I felt stabbing, piercing pains in my forearms and hands and I had to put him down immediately. For me, that was the moment that I had to admit that I needed help and could no longer hope that the problem would just fix itself.

So, I made an appointment for the GP the following day. I was so nervous going to that appointment, scared of the diagnosis, but also scared he'd dismiss it all and say it was in my head.

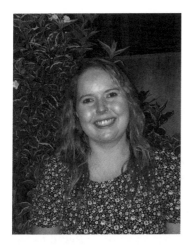

Breda Kane

I found myself crying as I was telling him my symptoms, finally letting all my fears and concerns out, thankfully he was wonderful.

He listened to it all, discussed that he felt it could be something rheumatic and that I needed blood tests as soon as possible. That week I went on sick leave, due to the pain and stiffness worsening, alongside feeling constantly exhausted with no energy. I got my bloods done, it showed an elevated CRP and ESR, but my rheumatoid factor was negative. My GP then referred me to a rheumatologist, for further investigations.

I was lucky enough to be able to go private for my rheumatology appointment, so only had to wait two weeks instead of two years. Those two weeks felt like a lifetime, I spent it googling so many different conditions, as my GP had mentioned what he thought it could be.

Thankfully as Christmas was just around the corner, I had something else to focus on. I did all my shopping and planning online trying to distract myself from worrying about my appointment.

On the day of the appointment, my consultant determined that I had rheumatoid arthritis, he wanted another set of blood tests, along with an x-ray of my hands and chest. I was to start on a course of steroids and then to see him again in six weeks.

I tried to stay positive, thinking how much worse a diagnosis I could've gotten. But my sister said the most amazing thing to me, when I told her it could be worse.

She said, 'It could be worse, but it's still shite', and that was exactly what I needed to hear.

I needed to be reminded that even though there are other conditions I could have gotten, that I was still allowed to feel devastated by this diagnosis. And I was devastated, as I have seen first-hand how challenging living with a chronic illness can be for a person.

The steroids helped reduce the pain, but they never made me feel like me again. I went back to work and only managed to work three shifts, before having to go off sick again. The second time was more upsetting than the first, as I started to wonder if I would ever be able to get back to work properly again. I went back to see the rheumatologist at the end of January, and he commenced me on a DMARD (disease-modifying anti-rheumatic drug), I was given a weaning course of steroids for 10 weeks and then back to see the consultant in 16 weeks.

For a short period, I was starting to feel good, I was able to return to work and was managing. I no longer did night shifts and I was only doing one shift at a time, no two days in a row or anything like that.

When I returned to work, I only had six weeks until annual leave and I remember being so proud of myself making it to that six-week mark without any sick leave, it felt like such an accomplishment.

Once I weaned off the steroids though, the pain started to return, but thanks to my new system of working my shifts, I at least managed to keep working.

In May 2018, I turned 30; I had such great plans, my boyfriend took me away for a few days to Fota Island, but unfortunately the pain and just a cramping/nausea feeling in my stomach ruled those few days. We powered through a bit and tried to make the most of it, but my plan of ringing in the midnight as I turned 30, with a cocktail in my hand, didn't happen. Instead I was upstairs asleep, purely exhausted from it all. And that's rheumatoid arthritis all over, at times it just takes away the little things from you, the ones that may mean the most.

I saw my consultant again at the end of May and he decided to increase my treatment and once again a weaning course of steroids to keep me going.

One of my close friends was getting married in the middle of June. I had always been a high-heeled shoe girl, I loved them; I probably had about 25 pairs of heels in my wardrobe. But I could no longer stand in a pair for more than two minutes, without terrible pain in my ankles and feet, and it broke my heart. I became obsessed with finding a pretty pair of flats to make up for this, but I couldn't find any as nice as the heels I would have worn.

It was such a trivial thing, nobody probably noticed my shoes and if they did, they probably took no heed, but to me it was horrendous, it was another thing arthritis had taken from me.

On the increased drug dose, my pain remained the same, the only change was that on the day of and day after I took it, I now felt terribly sick. I had to plan to be off the following day and couldn't really plan to do much in case I needed a bathroom. The glamorous life of trying to find medication that worked.

At the end of August, I once again headed off for my rheumatologist appointment, hopeful for a medication that will work. At this appointment, we agreed for me to start biologics, reduced the DMARD and another weaning dose of steroids. A month later, I was starting to wonder if it was working, as I was starting to feel better.

Unfortunately, though once I started to reduce the steroids the pain would come back. In November around the year mark, I was beginning to feel worse than ever, I was managing to keep working, but my days off were being spent completely exhausted and sore on the couch recovering from any activity. At this stage I was just getting fed up with it all, it was beginning to feel like a never-ending cycle of appointments, sick days, medications and pain.

My next rheumatologist appointment was early December, my boyfriend and I went to the appointment very fed up with the whole situation; my consultant decided to go over everything. We went back through all my original and current symptoms, and he examined me once again. He decided to do a full body MRI to make sure there was nothing else going on. The MRI was done mid-January and I was back to see the rheumatologist at the start of February.

The new plan was to start on a different biologic, along with the DMARD and to once again start on a weaning dose of steroids, this time the dose would be higher for longer. In the middle of April, I started to find that I was able to do a little more, I'd less pain and a bit more energy.

My boyfriend and my sister both commented that they noticed an improvement too. We had a planned holiday to Budapest, and I found that unlike previous holidays since my diagnosis, I was able to do more and stay up later, as I had more energy.

At the end of May, I went back to see the rheumatologist. My CRP was still up, but because I was feeling well and thinking the new treatment was working, it was agreed I would continue with this biologic for the moment and continue reducing my dose of steroids. By late July, I am now in the middle of another flare-up and currently off work, due to the pain and fatigue. I have spoken to my consultant and the plan is to now start on a new drug. I've been doing my research, know what to expect and all I can do is keep my fingers crossed and hope that this will be my miracle drug.

When I first got diagnosed, I had a few friends tell me 'Oh I know such and such with that and now they're doing well, completely back to themselves a year later.' And I really wanted that to be me.

I have since spoken to one of my friends about that, and we were saying people probably say the same about me at times. They see my Instagram or Facebook and see me out and about, not realising that half an hour after such a picture I was sitting in a corner as I needed a rest or that I was too sore or tired and had to go home.

I think that's what people need to remember. I never talk about or put up pictures of the days where I struggle to get out of bed in the morning due to pain, I don't talk about the fact that I haven't driven for longer than 30 minutes in nearly two years, people don't know the frustration I feel when I'm unable to hold a cup of tea for more than 30 seconds and there's only a handful of people who know about all the times I cry when I'm feeling lost and unsure if I will ever be able to manage this condition.

However, I don't want to be all negative, my life hasn't

stopped since my diagnosis. I have just finished a postgraduate degree in my specialist area, I'm still unsure how I managed it at times, but I did. And I recently got engaged, so I have that to look forward to, hopefully I'll be on a drug that works by that time.

So even though there are days where I'm in tears, 'cause I can't get out of bed or leave my apartment due to the pain and fatigue, there are plenty of other days that I get to go out and enjoy the world like I use to, just perhaps at a slower pace.

Anne Kelly

My mam always used to say that there is no difference between an egg cup and a 10-gallon barrel, for once both are full, they will overflow. Which is how I would describe my slow, but eventual coming to terms with my diagnosis of rheumatoid arthritis.

Ah yeah, the diagnosis itself is curiously deceptive and covers a multitude, because RA is actually a chronic autoimmune disease, which means that our immune systems have decided the we ourselves are actually the dreaded plague, the virus, the enemy it must fight so aggressively against. And, by God, does it fight against us!!

On 21 March 2018, I went to my doctor's surgery for the results of my blood tests, never ever suspecting for one moment that I would find myself in front of my GP, who almost had tears in his eyes, as he gave me the ominous news.

I had a very serious, incurable illness, called RA. My only reason for going to see him in the first place was because I thought the recent onslaught of a constant feeling of having flu, the pain in my hands, the stiffness in my neck and shoulders, the limp I'd developed in my right leg, etc., etc. were all just physical signs of the awful toll that grief, loss and bereavement were having on me.

Strangely enough, this date of my diagnosis is highly

significant, if not just downright cruel. Because, you see, it was exactly six months to the actual day, when, on 21 June 2017, my gorgeous, six-foot tall, madly vain, gym-bunny, youngest son, Laurence, had died very suddenly. He was 30 years and two months old. Yeah, strange that.

I was referred to Tallaght Hospital, rheumatology department, as an 'Urgent' case. It actually took eight months to get my first appointment. I was prescribed a DMARD (disease-modifying anti-rheumatic drug) and folic acid, and I went home and refused to take them.

I'd heard all the horror stories, and no, I was going to fight this with natural means. Until, two weeks later, on a Friday, I woke up, unable to move and in sheer agony. Yep, welcome to the flare from the Seventh Circle of Hell.

As luck would have it, I had a rheumy appointment on the Monday morning and I shuffled up there, blind with the pain. I was also dreading telling them I had not taken the prescribed meds, but I must have looked so pitiful to the amazing rheumy team, that they immediately gave me the most wonderful, merciful steroid injection and switched me to the DMARD injections weekly. Bless their hearts. I was human again. And, if they had told me to inject cat pee, I would have. Lesson learned.

I now take my injection every Monday and while it subdues the pain, it does not totally eliminate it, and sometimes I really struggle. There is NO family history of RA, and until my son's death, I had been mostly as healthy as a trout. The fact that I received my diagnosis on the sixth month anniversary makes it impossible for me to believe there is not a correlation between the onset of autoimmune disease and severe shock and trauma. Yeah, strange that.

This is my RA story ... and ... I'm sticking to it!

Naomi Kelly

Have you ever heard someone say, 'I have this banging headache that I can't seem to get rid of', despite the fact that they took two painkillers? That's the only way I can describe rheumatoid arthritis.

People automatically associate this disease with an older generation, as I would have too. But this is not the case. I was 29 when I was diagnosed, had been sick for nearly a year with a cold, no energy, unable to even carry the laundry basket up the stairs without struggling to catch my breath.

This was someone who walked 6k most days, went to the gym four mornings a week and didn't even know the sofa was uncomfortable because she never sat on it!

I went to the doctor who did some blood tests and, when I got the call, was told in a very matter of fact fashion, 'You have rheumatoid arthritis, you will be sent a letter for the early detection clinic in Tallaght.'

You're not quite sure how to respond. It doesn't seem quite real and not having any knowledge of the condition, it seemed easy to ignore until the appointment in the clinic...

Sitting in the waiting room, alone and staring at an artist's impression of the condition, surrounded by older patients, thinking I don't belong here. That artist impression of disfigured hands nearly on fire comes to me every time I close my eyes.

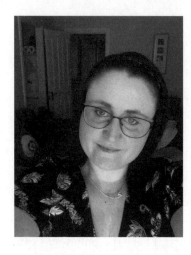

Naomi Kelly

Sitting in the doctor's room; listening to an unfamiliar language; terms you don't know or don't want to have to understand; going to get x-rays and bloods; walking to your car, your head spinning, with the nurse's words in your head, 'I would hate this condition.'

You drive to work and tears stream down your face, because you are frightened of this thing that's taking over your body. Little do you know that with those little words, your whole world will change.

Sometimes you wish that you had cancer, because that can be cured or will kill you, rather than being trapped in this arthritis limbo.

With those words, 'You have rheumatoid arthritis' my life changed. My now ex-partner of 13 years couldn't deal with the depression that sent me to bed or me talking about what the illness would mean for our future. Your body changed, the medications made me put on weight, the pain meant I couldn't exercise as much, I felt trapped, useless and unwanted.

You look in the mirror and you don't see you. This, I

think, is the hardest thing to accept, that there was a pre-diagnosis you and there is a post-diagnosis you. You have to adjust to this new you and I plead with anyone reading this to ask for help, to talk openly and honestly about how tired you are or how much pain you're in. To ask for help and know that you are not alone. There are others out there who are fighting the same fight as you and while no fight is the same, you will march on.

There will be hard days and harder days, lonely days, especially when life becomes a cycle of clinics, x-rays, steroid injections, doctors who will ask questions, that you will want to scream at because they don't understand, because they don't walk in your shoes.

Take a breath, you will get through this. Reward yourself on the good days and let yourself rest on the bad days.

Be prepared for 'the look' from people, like you've told them you have leprosy, that if they touch you, they will catch it. They just don't understand. You're a fighter though, don't let them disarm you or run you down; it will hurt, but you will get back up and keep going because you have no choice. Find someone you can talk to.

I have attended talk therapy for five years since I was diagnosed, became single, lost my house and had to start life all over again. Talking helps.

Life now is different, it's definitely not the one I dreamed of or planned for. The road has taken a different direction with more hills, sometimes than I have the energy to climb. On those days I sit and look at the view.

Life will go on after this diagnosis, I have a job I love, I travel, I date (when someone swipes right). I have lost friends and relationships because of my condition, but I have found amazing people (who understand I can be very cranky with pain), who provide a support system that I couldn't manage without. I have a family who care for and love me; a fur baby who keeps me active and moving, who provides unconditional love and cuddles on those bad days.

Listen to your body, rest, even if it's just having a shower that has made you tired. Feel free to grieve and cry for you – but I hope you fall in love with you again too, and see that you are not this condition, but you are just you.

Jason Kerins

I'm from Castleisland, Co. Kerry and was diagnosed with rheumatoid arthritis and psoriatic arthritis in 2014, when I was 34. I was a welder, fitter/fabricator, used to also look after the family farm (with my dad's help), enjoyed road running and ran marathons for fun. Married with two boys, I had to find time for them, so, to put it simply, I was always rushing and pushed for time every day.

The turning point in my life came when I received a call from the hospital to have some troublesome veins removed from my leg. These had become an issue after a road traffic accident in 2000.

Although the operation went very well, the vein was massive and there was a big opening in my hip where the vein was pulled from, which took longer than expected to heal and caused a lot of discomfort.

Stress levels were high around that time; a family member had passed away and I was doing a part-time agriculture course.

I didn't have any symptoms at that time, but when I started back training, I had pains in my knees, which I didn't take too much notice of. Being a distance runner, pains and twinges are common, but at the same time, something didn't feel right.

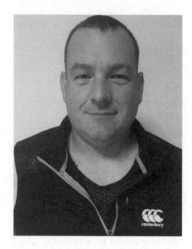

Jason Kerins

I wasn't able to make progress, I tried different things, but just couldn't get going. As time went on, the pains got worse and moved to my lower back. I was now really struggling, physically and mentally.

I had gone from working full-time and running on average between 60-80 miles a week to my kids having to help me get dressed in the morning. I couldn't raise my leg over the shower tray, couldn't pick anything up off the ground; I found myself in a place I was never in before.

It was the lowest point in my life; no running, work hurt, and everything was a struggle.

My wife, Jillian, was fantastic, she was always there for me and could see when I was feeling down. She often took the kids for a drive to leave me alone in the house. On those days, I would go back to bed, curled in a ball with the sheets pulled up and either slept or started to cry, out of sheer frustration with what was happening to me.

My own doctor was fantastic, but had limited treatment options available. With the rheumatology waiting list being so long, it took ages to be called.

When I finally got to see a rheumatologist, being told 'I'll look after you' gave me some hope and I was started on treatment, going quickly from a DMARD (disease-modifying anti-rheumatic drug) to a biologic.

By this time, I was unable to commit to work. After a few weeks on the biologic, the pain had started to ease off and I began to feel normal again. Although I knew that I would never get back to how I used to be, being pain-free was as good a gift as any.

One of the consequences of the tablets and steroids was that the weight piled on. It felt like a snowflake landing on a mountain top, rolling down the side, getting bigger and gaining momentum. I tried so hard, but no matter what I did, the scales only went one way.

Having been sleep-deprived for years – it's very hard to feel good about yourself when you're tired and fatigued – five years on, and I'm finally getting some proper rest.

That's made a big difference, my mood is happier, I'm back walking – in fact, I started running last week, the first time since 2014. I know I will never run a marathon again, but it won't stop me trying. My aim is to pin on a race number again, not this year but in 2020 hopefully for a 10k.

As long as the arthritis is at bay, the future is bright.

Claire Kinneavy

The words 'rheumatology department' were very noticeable as I took a short cut through St James's Hospital in the late 1970s. I was a student home economics teacher and often stayed nearby at my sister's place. I hadn't a clue what rheumatology meant or indeed how familiar it would become a few years later!

I was diagnosed with severe rheumatoid arthritis when I was just 24 years old. A new mum, I was on maternity leave from work, happily caring for my little son. I had a trouble-free pregnancy and was looking forward to getting back to work.

Instead, I noticed increasing fatigue, loss of strength and joint stiffness! This was followed by severe and fleeting joint pains in my hands, wrists, elbows, shoulders, feet and knees.

The pain was intense and luckily my GP recognised RA and immediately referred me to a rheumatologist. My GP was very sensitive and conveyed the seriousness of my diagnosis in a kind and caring voice without alarming me unduly. He reassured me just as quickly that treatments had improved a lot and that research was promising!

This was 1982 and the gold injections I was likely to start on had become more refined and effective and research was advancing nicely he told me.

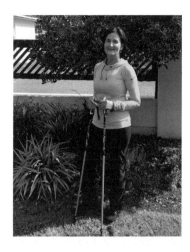

Claire Kinneavy

I believed and put my trust in him and my optimistic nature helped me to visualise an improvement. More importantly I visualised even better drugs and a cure in my lifetime!

My baby was only 10 weeks old when I received the unwelcome diagnosis in hospital! Perhaps it was a coincidence, but I was sharing a room with an elderly lady who had very severe rheumatoid arthritis. She was very debilitated, slept on a sheepskin rug and could only walk slowly with a walking frame.

Naturally I was scared that I might become so disabled, but I plucked up the courage to ask for some helpful tips.

I can only remember one very important message, 'Don't stop doing ANYTHING!' She was still enjoying some embroidery to pass the time in hospital and I have never forgotten her and her determination.

I had conversations in my head about how I might cope with this incurable disease, which required medications with side effects, constant vigilance and adjustments. I reassured myself that the disease was physical in nature and preferable to mental ill health. I knew that the disease could cause havoc, so I vowed to do three things.

1) I promised myself that I would work hard to try and stay as well as I could by taking the medications, being vigilant about side effects, keeping appointments and getting blood tests.

2) Always visualise a good outcome and wonderful new medicines on the horizon.

3) While it was a disease with lots of physical manifestations, I promised to try and focus on the positives in order to maintain a good frame of mind. I vowed that if I couldn't continue in paid employment, I would try and do some voluntary work with a patient organisation.

Fast forward over three years, I had returned to work and was expecting my second child and had a very easy pregnancy. After my daughter was born, I had another severe flare-up of the disease.

It took quite a while for the rheumatologist to get the disease under control, but I found a wonderful physiotherapist who taught me how to cope with the joint swellings, stiffness and pain. She also taught me how to put my joints through full range of motion and encouraged me to attend the rheumatology services at Harold's Cross.

I retired from my full-time job, as there was quite a lot of damage to my hands, wrists and elbows. I became used to having joint injections to ease pain and remove excess fluid by always ensuring I didn't look at the needle and visualising a good result!

Disappointed as I was to finish work, I found it easier when I could no longer recognise the students in uniform and enjoyed looking after the children. I had fun taking them to swimming lessons, adventure centres and playgrounds and took rest while they were at school. Hospital stays allowed them the opportunity to visit and become close to their cousins and this was an additional benefit as family rowed in to help.

Medication had not prevented some permanent joint damage, but I remained upbeat and tried to keep up with everyone else. A branch of Arthritis Ireland had started in Co. Kildare in 1986 and this coincided with my retirement. I joined the committee and had some nice opportunities to meet new people in the community.

I was open and honest about my disease and people were often surprised that I was SO young to have arthritis. 'Cures' were offered and suggested by well-meaning friends and acquaintances and I tried them all! I travelled distances and spent lots of money to try homeopathy, herbalism, exclusion diets, supplementary nutrients, bio energy, prayer meetings, potions and lotions.

Somehow the notion that I was so young and that 'cures' were available made me feel GUILTY! I was still full of HOPE! I had become familiar with the blood tests, x-rays and terminology used when talking to the health professionals and learned to observe the signs of active disease. I could tell that the cures were not working and the medications not preventing damage and I became AFRAID for the first time!

A visit to an upper limb specialist confirmed that there was permanent damage to my hands, wrists and elbow. It had taken 10 years for me to become really upset and SAD. I couldn't believe that I needed an elbow replacement at 35. I had reached rock bottom! The elbow replacement was very successful, but the rehabilitation period afterwards was quite tough and required lots of physiotherapy.

Fortunately, the Arthritis Ireland self-management

programme was being piloted in Ireland and I paid £10 to do the six-week programme. It was the best money I'd spent, as I found it extremely helpful.

No one had explained the cycle of pain to me heretofore and it really helped me to get it all into perspective! In addition, I learned about the importance of using skills such as positive thinking, problem solving, setting goals and good communication and how natural it is to feel sad or feel loss when living with arthritis. It was also a great opportunity to meet others with arthritis.

Shortly afterwards I trained as a self-management leader and enjoyed delivering the programme with a co-leader. I became more involved with Arthritis Ireland and began to organise educational and exercise events in my local area with other committee members. I joined a leisure centre and started enjoying aqua aerobics. I also tried yoga, dance and pilates classes. I became a lot less isolated and felt more involved in community life.

Keeping upbeat and hopeful is really crucial, but it is equally important to acknowledge the EMOTIONAL PAIN. It was possibly more difficult to deal with than the physical pain. My GP was very supportive and I acknowledged and offloaded all the feelings to him and to a professional counsellor. It didn't take long to fill up my emotional tank again with their help and that of family and friends.

I resolved to become a bit kinder to myself by purchasing lots of useful gadgets and got help with heavy housework. Over the next decade I had some more surgery including knuckle replacements and lots of medication adjustments until the advent of newer biologic drugs. Halleluiah!

The first biologic drug prescribed was delivered via an infusion in hospital. It worked much better than the DMARDs (disease-modifying anti-rheumatic drugs) on their own. One benefit of having the treatment in hospital was that I had the opportunity to meet other people living with arthritis and this was really beneficial.

Within weeks I noticed less fatigue, pain and swellings. My knees were less swollen and I didn't need joint injections for a long time. I was delighted as I felt more like my old self. I remained on this drug for a couple of years when a self-injecting drug was introduced to my treatment plan. I was apprehensive about injecting myself, but quickly got used to it and my hands were better able to handle the syringe. Fortunately for me, this drug worked extremely well and I looked forward to taking the medication weekly.

I participated in a physiotherapy-led exercise study at Harold's Cross specifically designed for people with RA on biologic medication and really enjoyed it. I attended several weeks of circuit training and this motivated me to try and find better opportunities to exercise and to problem solve around supportive footwear.

Ten years ago, I was involved in organising a local pilot Nordic walking programme for people with arthritis and have not looked back! The poles help me to mobilise my joints in preparation for walking and I've noticed a steady improvement in overall strength and fitness. It has also had additional benefit of helping to maintain bone density and meet new friends.

Six years ago, I had surgery on both feet to help with pain relief and correct hammer toes, etc. The rehabilitation period was lengthy and tough, but most worthwhile! I can now find shoes that are more fashionable and have a lot less pain.

As I had visualised and hoped over three decades earlier, my disease activity is now extremely low and blood tests confirm there is virtually no inflammation! I get four infusions yearly and take a DMARD daily. This is an even better combination of drugs for me. I rarely need extra painkillers unless I've overdone it!

I am extremely grateful that so much research has been carried out in my lifetime and that there are so many very effective drugs available. I am grateful too for an excellent healthcare team, patient organisation, family and friends. I am proud to be part of an arthritis community and consider any operation scars as imaginary war medals. I continue to experiment with exercise activities which keeps me mentally and physically fit. I also use all the coping skills I have learned to solve any problems that arise. I am really enjoying life and 'Living well with arthritis'!

Ger Kirrane

I am 40 years of age and have been living with rheumatoid arthritis for over five years now.

I was always a very active person. In my 20s, I played Gaelic football at senior level, played to a handicap of four in golf and played music professionally. In my early 30s, I worked full-time, commuting 100 miles a day to work, while playing music professionally most evenings during the week. I loved being on the go and keeping busy. Being active was part of my daily routine and I took it for granted.

In the summer of 2014, I started getting regular pain in my knees and shoulders, which I just put down to being tired. It would last several days and then clear up. After a couple of months, I decided to go to my GP to get it checked out. I expected to be told to rest and that it would be back to normal soon.

Upon examination, my doctor suggested doing some blood tests to check my rheumatoid factor. This was the first time I ever heard the word 'rheumatoid'. Within a couple of days, she confirmed that I had RA. My first thought was 'no, there's a mistake here', sure arthritis is an illness that only old men get! She referred me to a specialist, who later explained to me what was happening to my body and why I felt pain in my joints.

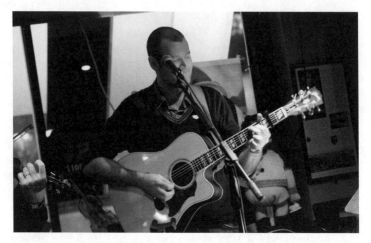

Ger Kirrane

By the time I had met him four weeks later, I was getting pain in my knees, shoulders, hands, wrists, and my energy levels were very low. His first plan of action was to put me on a disease-modifying drug (DMARD). It would decrease the pain and swelling from my arthritis and because I was diagnosed at a relatively young age, it should prevent joint damage, and reduce the risk of long-term disability.

Within a few months of being diagnosed I attended a 'Living Well with Arthritis' course that ran over six weeks, one evening a week. It was very informative, but also quite frightening. I was the newcomer to the RA family, so my symptoms weren't as bad as some other people. I could still do most things at this stage, while the person next to me couldn't open a bottle cap or hold a mug of tea in their hand. In my innocence I thought that will never happen to me, sure I've got this early!

As the months went on, I started noticing small differences in my ability to perform normal everyday tasks. Getting up out of bed became a struggle, putting on my clothes hurt a little, driving the car caused pain in my knees and lying on the couch when I was tired caused my knees to sporadically jerk. Watching this slowly happen to my body was a frightening experience and really worried me. The more I stressed about it though, the more pain and discomfort I felt.

The main difference I noticed during the first 12 months was that my energy levels were decreasing rapidly. During the second year I started to feel no benefit from the medication and was getting pain injections to get me through each month. My body had become immune to it.

Following my next consultation, we decided to change to another medication, a biologic, which was administered through an infusion every six weeks. My wife and I were trying for a family, so I had to avoid certain medications.

I have been on this treatment for over three years now. In addition to the infusion, I also take a daily tablet, which works alongside it, to try to keep the inflammation down.

Having an illness such as RA can be very challenging. On a good day, I can wake up and convince myself that I don't have it. I try to go about my normal day with approximately 60% of my energy level, but unfortunately, it's not long before my body reminds me of my illness.

A bad day is a horrible experience. I wake up extremely tired, get out of bed in pain and feel like I'm dragging my body around after me. Every task is a struggle. On days like this, you find it very difficult to find happiness or satisfaction in anything. I get angry and pissed off with the world. Why did I get this? I'm a good person I don't deserve this!

As I've experienced the bad days many times over the last few years, I am trying to develop a level of acceptance around it. Okay, it's a bad day, but what good can I make from it – I'll try to accept that today will be a tough day and tonight I'll have a hot bath to ease my joints and maybe watch Netflix on my iPad.

The term 'fake it to make it' comes to mind. Another way I try to deal with the pain is to find gratitude in what I *can* do and try to imagine someone else who is in a worst place, both physically and mentally, to me.

Living with this illness is a rollercoaster – you're up and you're down but hopefully with the right medication and treatment, you will have more ups than downs.

In the early days of living with this illness, I realised that there was a huge amount of information out there about all the different ways that people treat RA. Everyone I spoke to had a different 'cure' – cod liver oil, black cherry juice, cider vinegar, add ginger to your meals, copper soles in your shoes, copper bracelets, short walks, running on the beach, swimming in the sea, the list goes on. I have tried them all.

In 2016, I spent over €3,000 on a range of alternative treatments – acupuncture, bio-energy, holistic massages, counselling sessions, consults with kinesiologists, Chinese medicine treatments – trying to find the magic cure to get rid of this illness.

A tough part of my journey with RA has been dealing with the mental side of it. A couple of years ago when I was having more bad days than good on a regular basis, I struggled to deal with it. Within a two-week period I had to cancel going to a good friend's wedding and cancel attending another family occasion, I had to cancel two wedding bookings that I was due to play and the final straw for me was when I had to cancel playing a gig with a very famous UK band that I grew up listening to.

A group I played with were lined up to support them at a large festival in the south of Ireland. My friends had booked to come along, the weather was due to be fantastic and I couldn't wait to get on stage with them.

Two days before the gig, my pains had gotten so bad that I had to make a call to the band and drop out. It broke my heart and after the call I sat and cried for a good hour. All the frustration and sadness of having this disease came out that morning. It was beating me, and I had had enough.

Later that morning, I decided to make a call to a counselling service and arranged some sessions for the coming weeks. I had to talk this out with someone. It wouldn't fix my pain, but it might help me come to terms with it. I attended over a dozen sessions and it did help me find some acceptance that I had this illness and I had to manage it every day. It was my responsibility to manage this.

These days I try my best to have some time for myself during the week, whether that be a counselling session, a walk, a bath, listening to music or coffee and a book. The effect of long working days that include several hours driving is taking its toll on my body. If I don't slow down every few days and take care of myself, then I will feel pain very quickly.

In the last couple of years, I have noticed some things that trigger my pains and I try to monitor them as much as possible – sleep, driving, stress and diet. Without eight hours sleep, my body shuts down. For many years I lived off three or four hours when I worked and played music in the evenings. Now if I can't or don't sleep at night, I will pay the price in the morning. I face the next day with little or no energy. Weekends are important for me now to catch up on missed sleep during the week.

Driving my car causes me a lot of pain. What is a simple task for many people, of holding the wheel with both hands, feels like a workout in the gym to me. An hour in the car feels like I've been lifting weights. Having my knees, particularly my right one, in a held position moving up and down on the accelerator causes me pain both in that moment and for a few hours after I have stopped driving. Soon I will have to change my job as my body can't continue to be put through this pain for much longer.

Stress and diet are also triggers for the symptoms. Today I try to keep my stress levels down as much as possible and eat as healthily as possible. The main exercise I can do these days is walking and I try to get as many walks in during the week as possible.

It's a hard thing trying to describe to someone how you feel living with RA. I can put on a suit and go to work and by looking at me you wouldn't think anything was wrong. I can be friendly, smile and be part of the team. Unfortunately, underneath that suit and smile is a person who is broken and sad. I have stopped trying to explain to people about the pain levels, because they will never know unless they have it themselves. While people are trying to be nice and asking how you are, the only way they would appreciate what I'm going through is if they had this illness themselves for a month.

My life today is about managing this pain and trying to make the best out of each day. Now and again I get glimpses of the old me. Last week I was golfing and for a while I felt like my 20-year-old self. I picked up three birdies in six holes on the front nine, had confidence in myself and my game, but on the back nine the pain and tiredness kicked in and I no longer wanted to be out there. It was like the switch was turned off and suddenly I didn't want to play anymore.

At least once a week I leave the office or go somewhere quiet for a few minutes to have a cry with the pain I feel and unless you have the illness, you can't understand how frustrating and upsetting it can be. Behind the smile and mask that I put on to the outside world, underneath I often feel broken and lost.

Today as I write this, it is a relatively good day. I am tired, have pain in my shoulders, knees and neck and have about 50-60% energy levels. This is as good as it gets. I need to make the most of out today because I don't know what tomorrow will bring. Maybe it will be different, and I'll be free of this illness once and for all. Maybe not, but where there's life, there's hope!

Denise Lowe

I was diagnosed with rheumatoid arthritis in summer 2011. It hit me like a bolt of lightning and there are still days when I find it hard to accept that I have this disease. I felt why was this happening to me, it's not fair and I became highly anxious and worried about my future..

My diagnosis came as a relief though, as the pain I was in prior to this was chronic and unexplained. I was constantly shuffling around on a swollen ankle or knee, or unable to lift my arm which had felt like it had been broken. My children were still very young too, so every day was such a challenge.

When I was diagnosed, my rheumatologist was very helpful, explained my condition, the medication I would be taking, but it was all too much on that day. Although he was talking, I was no longer taking in what he was saying; my world was crashing down around me.

How was I going to cope with this for life, the pain, the uncertainty and to that end, I was grieving for myself and it took time for that sadness to subside.

In the months that followed, I began to slowly pick myself up and tried to get as much information as I could on the condition, I reached out to some friends who had also been diagnosed to see how they managed the disease.

It was great to find people who completely understood

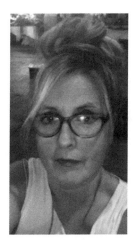

Denise Lowe

your pain, because often people don't understand just how hard it is to cope with the invisible pain of RA. The medication I'm on has helped me greatly with managing pain and swelling, my only qualm about the medication is the effect it has on my liver (I have liver checks annually now), but it definitely works in terms of my pain management and allows me for the most part to have a full and active life.

Another element of this disease is the effect that RA has on our mental health, I often find I'm depressed and tired and everything is an effort. When joint pain flares-up there is the endless cycle of no exercise for maybe weeks on end, which leads to feeling more depressed, coping with pain and fatigue.

In the end it comes down to managing this disease as best you can, as with anything, eating well and exercise will help, taking the medications you are prescribed and getting support from family, friends and support systems like Arthritis Ireland who offer great advice and information to arthritis sufferers.

I found Arthritis Ireland particularly helpful when first diagnosed as this is a scary time when you realise you have a lifelong illness and you need to have support systems in place and get as much information and help as you can.

As I said at the beginning, there are days I find it hard to accept my disease, but for the most part I try to live my best life and manage RA with all the supports offered to me.

RA does not define the person you are; seek the supports you need to help you live your best life.

Des McGuinness

My experience of having RA began suddenly one morning in February 2017, when I was unable to get out of bed, dress or tie my laces without my wife's assistance. My hands had become claw-like and it was painful to make a fist. The transition from being an active, healthy 68-year-old guy to one that was aching, stiff and unable to move seemed to have happened overnight.

Upon examination, my GP diagnosed polymyology arthritis (PMR) and prescribed a course of steroids, but when the stiffness spread from my pelvic collar to my feet, neck and shoulders, alongside a heightened sense of fatigue and crankiness, I was referred to a consultant who diagnosed rheumatoid arthritis in March 2017 and prescribed a DMARD (disease-modifying anti-rheumatic drug).

Talking to friends, I received advice to check out the role of the Mediterranean diet and regular exercise in the well-being of patients with RA. I also checked out websites run by Arthritis Ireland, the Mayo Clinic, the NHS, etc. where I learnt that while there is little medical research to support the benefits of alternative remedies, it made sense to me to avoid foods and drink that may cause inflammation and may put a strain on the digestive system. As a family we were already eating a diet fairly close to the Mediterranean one, including

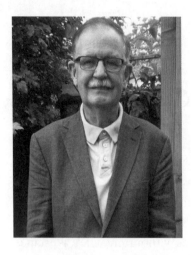

Des McGuinness

oily fish, fruit and vegetables and baking our own oat bread.

Then in September 2017 I was diagnosed with pneumonia, was hospitalised and taken off the DMARD, raising questions as to its impact on my immune system and, more particularly, a possible vulnerability to chest infections due to having had pulmonary TB as a young man. My rheumatologist subsequently changed my medication to a different DMARD and thankfully all is going well, with my blood markers at their lowest level since I was first diagnosed with RA.

Attending a Living Well with Arthritis course in 2019 provided me with the opportunity to learn from others who are living with various degrees of arthritic pain and to reflect on the best ways to live with RA guided by a personal action plan.

So, what are the lessons that I have learnt about living with rheumatoid arthritis?

- The importance of having a good GP and consultant and listening to them. Going to my GP promptly after the onset of sudden stiffness;

- Having the love and support of family members;
- Communicating my feelings to my partner and listening to her feedback;
- Taking responsibility for my own diet and exercise;
- Walking for at least 30 minutes five times a week;
- Limiting daytime naps to 30 minutes by setting a clock/timer alarm;
- Being wary of the claims of alternative medicines and supplements in the treatment of RA;
- Talking to other RA sufferers, but keeping the 'organ recital' short;
- Keeping a diary from the time I was diagnosed with RA;
- Keeping informed about developments in the treatment of RA.

While RA is a chronic autoimmune condition and medical intervention is essential, for me accepting the situation, keeping on the move, having a positive mental attitude and being thankful that it is not too severe has been very helpful to my well-being, as indeed is the love and solidarity of family and friends.

Maryanne Murphy-Lyons

As I sit down to start writing my story of living with rheumatoid arthritis, it stirs up old anxieties and fears I used to have about living with RA. So I feel I should almost start this story like it will end and that is that I am now living well with rheumatoid arthritis, but the living well element did take time for various reasons.

The birth of our third child in October 2015 was a very exciting time for my husband Niall and I; our little boy Harry was welcomed adoringly into our family by our two other children James and Sarah, who were aged six and two respectively.

Harry was a great baby, he was instantly very good at breastfeeding and sleeping, almost perfect! Unfortunately, within four to six weeks of Harry's birth, I started to feel unwell. While I was familiar with the usual post-partum aches and pains and tiredness that are common with a newborn baby, this was different and almost unrelenting.

Harry was approximately four weeks old when I first noticed that I seemed to be very stiff, especially getting out of bed in the morning. Every day I was noticing something different, swollen knee, ankle, my hands were feeling hot and swollen. I was noticing the stiffness was getting worse and increasing every day at an alarming rate.

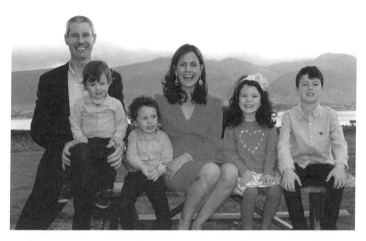

Maryanne Murphy-Lyons pictured (l-r) with her husband Niall, Samuel, Harry, Sarah and James

Around this time, I also developed a nasty sinus infection and little Harry was also overdue his six-week check-up. I made an appointment with my GP and I mentioned that I was feeling unwell. He was extremely attentive and showed great care to me as I cried, explaining that I was feeling so awful and was struggling with lifting and holding Harry. He carefully examined my hot swollen joints and he did a full set of bloods, including testing me for the rheumatoid factor. I didn't understand why he was testing me for the rheumatoid factor at that time. He prescribed antibiotics for my sinus infection and medication for the pain in my joints.

My GP rang me a few days later that my blood results were clear and that the rheumatoid factor was negative and to see how I was feeling. My sinus infection was much better, but my symptoms of hot, painful, swollen joints and joint stiffness continued. My GP said to come back to him in one week, which I did. It was almost Christmas and l was feeling more and more anxious and in a lot of pain.

I will never forget that consultation with my GP, and looking back at it now, he was correct in everything he said. He told me that he felt I was developing seronegative arthritis and that I needed to see a rheumatologist after Christmas.

He advised me that I would need good coping skills and a positive mental attitude in the coming weeks. He commenced me on a course of steroids to reduce the inflammation in my joints and improve my joint stiffness.

In the following weeks, lots of family and friends came to help me manage baby Harry and my other two children. I consulted with various alternative therapists to try alleviate my symptoms, acupuncture, reflexology, osteopathy to name a few! Indeed more than one person suggested to me that stopping breastfeeding would help my joints and alleviate my symptoms.

Thankfully, I did not do this. I consulted with Dr Jack Newman, a world-famous expert in Canada on breastfeeding, who absolutely reassured me that I could continue breastfeeding, despite my joint pain and stiffness.

I started to google more on seronegative arthritis and started to realise that my GP was worried I had rheumatoid arthritis. I reassured myself that this was not the case as my blood test was negative and I had no family history of RA.

I became determined not to have rheumatoid arthritis!

Nonetheless, I was struggling to manage the pain and stiffness in my joints, while looking after Harry and my other two children.

My appointment with a rheumatologist a few weeks later confirmed exactly what my GP had suggested to me, that I had developed rheumatoid arthritis. He explained that the rheumatoid factor could be negative; I did not know that you do not need to have a family history of RA to develop it. The rheumatologist also explained to me that women are two to three times as likely as men to develop RA and that post-partum onset is not uncommon.

Reassuringly, he advised me that I could continue breastfeeding. He prescribed medication for me called a DMARD (disease-modifying anti-rheumatic drug).

I found the following weeks very difficult, as I tried to accept that I had RA. I continued to try lots of alternative therapies and alternative diets and I didn't start the medication that was recommended.

I know now that this is not advisable and there is little scientific evidence to support the effectiveness of alternatives like herbs or acupuncture and strict diets for RA. I found it difficult to cope and worried so much all the time about my future living with this condition.

I sought an opinion of another rheumatologist during this time and he confirmed what my GP and the first rheumatologist advised that about my post-partum onset RA. I agreed after this consultation to commence the recommended medication and a course of short-term steroids. During this period of time, we discovered to our surprise and delight that, we were having another baby.

Pregnancy affects people with autoimmune disease differently and RA is no exception to this. Many people enjoy full periods of disease remission during pregnancy. My symptoms improved greatly during my early pregnancy and I felt better than I had in months! However, remission from my RA did not last long and my symptoms slowly started to return at around 25/30 weeks pregnant.

My fears and anxieties about RA caused a lot of distress to me at this time and I was very worried about having another baby and coping with the pain and stiffness and a post-partum flare-up. While pregnancy can give short-term remission from active disease in RA, post-partum flare-ups are very common.

During this time, I was referred to Prof. Doug Veale and Louise Moore, advance nurse practitioner in rheumatology in Our Lady's Hospice Harold's Cross, who have a special interest in rheumatology and reproductive health. This referral was a very important part of me now living well and understanding rheumatoid arthritis.

I was 30 weeks pregnant and was very worried about coping with another new baby and RA. However, with some education and consultation with Louise Moore, I was reassured that post-partum flare-ups can be very well managed and I found reassurance that she would be in touch me four to six weeks after my baby's birth. My RA symptoms were managed with a low dose steroid for the rest of my pregnancy.

Samuel was born just in time for Christmas on 18 December 2016; we came home to a very busy, excited house. We had a wonderful Christmas with our little new baby boy.

However, as expected within four to six weeks of Samuel's birth, I started to have a post-partum flare-up. Around this time, Louise contacted me and together we made a plan to manage my symptoms; this meant increasing my medication.

I was in a much better place psychologically this time as I had the support I needed and I was not in as much pain due to the medication. I was only taking steroids at this time which offered a temporary relief from RA symptoms and are not a long-term solution to managing RA.

When Samuel was about five months, I was finished breastfeeding him and my symptoms of RA were still active. The following eight to nine months were difficult, as I tried various combinations of medication to manage my RA. There are a number of different medications available to manage RA and it can be trial and error to find the right combination. It can also take a number of months to see the benefit of the medications.

Unfortunately, side effects are also common and it is a careful balance of medication and side effects that make the process of finding the correct medication important. What I have learned from that process as a patient is that you must be compliant and cooperative and be an active participant in your own care.

This is something that took me a while to learn, as I was not the most compliant patient and this did not help managing my RA. Keeping a diary of your symptoms, medication benefits and side effects all assist your doctor/nurse to provide you with the best care possible. I also found during this time that it is important to develop a relationship with your pharmacist, as they are another source of information and support.

I have always been a very active person and was used to exercising, but I started exercising more frequently as I found it helped my joint stiffness and also helped my coping skills. After a number of months and a couple of different medication changes, a suitable medication was found that suited me and alleviated my symptoms with minimal side effects.

I was able to slowly wean-off my steroids. During this period, I also attended other professionals such as a physiotherapist and occupational therapist. This was also a very important step for me, they taught me invaluable skills and shared great insights with me on managing pain, stress and fatigue, all common and reoccurring symptoms of RA.

As I learnt more about RA, I grew more confident in managing my life with the condition, as opposed to viewing it as something separate. Becoming an active participant in your own care is very important and, in my view, it has been one of the key factors in me living well with RA.

It does take some energy and emotional management and I do still get 'tired' of RA, but I no longer fear it like I did three years ago and when I am in periods of pain or fatigue I can recognise these symptoms and self-manage them.

Becoming an active participant as opposed to a passive recipient in my own care gave me the confidence to learn my self-management skills. Exercise, living a healthy, balanced, but busy life with work and four young children and my RA are the norm for me now!

RA no longer impacts my life in the way it used to, it is now just part of my life.

Sarah Murray

I'm 18 years old and I was diagnosed with RA when I was 16 in November 2017. Over the past year and a half, I've had many ups and downs when it has come to my condition.

We've had the big victories of me getting a few steroid injections and the smaller victories of me going a full day without taking painkillers! There have also been some losses along the way, some bigger than others like when I realised my medication wasn't working or less monumental, when I had to miss almost two weeks of school at the start of sixth year.

There have been difficult moments and I have no doubt that there will continue to be more, but I've also gained a lot of insight from living with this condition.

The idea that I might have rheumatoid arthritis came about when I went to the GP about a sinus infection. Just as I was leaving, I happened to mention my crooked left elbow, which had been stuck at a 150° angle since I was 14. Of course, it was pretty uncomfortable, but oddly enough, I didn't think much of it.

Before I knew where I was, I was in Crumlin hospital and giving a rheumatologist details of my history with joint pain and other odd symptoms. I told her about the spontaneous rashes I always got when I was little, the on and off pains in

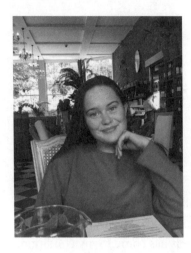
Sarah Murray

my 'dodgy' knees, my 'tricky tummy,' my tiredness, my achy back and finally, the crooked elbow.

All the while the rheumatologist sat opposite me, like Leonardo de Vinci, painting the art piece that is my rheumatoid arthritis. It had begun. It was at this moment that I was 100% sure that things were about to change.

Shortly after this, I had my first steroid injection in my elbow. Then I was put on a medication, which involved a weekly self-administered injection and took a bit of getting used to. I was on this drug for 12 weeks before we came to the conclusion that it was not working.

It was within this period that I had my first recognised flare-up. This was when I truly came to understand the extremity of my illness and the impact it was going to have on my life.

I was exhausted all the time and almost every joint in my body hurt constantly. It was really difficult because I was only 17 at this time but suddenly, I missed out on concerts and parties, because I just wasn't up for them. I've learned to monitor and manage my flares a lot better now. I have learned not to become overwhelmed with sadness when I have to miss something because I'm too sick, but I've also learned to not succumb to this illness and to not let it control every aspect of my life.

I have yet to find a medication that works for me and so, I've always found the side effects that come with the injections hard to deal with, because I'm not reaping the benefits of the medication. The DMARD (disease-modifying anti-rheumatic drug) had the worst side effects, which had a hugely negative impact on my life and well-being. Before I knew where I was, I was taking daily naps as a result of the fatigue, I was sick all the time due to my suppressed immune system, I couldn't eat anything other than white carbs because everything else made me sick and little bits of my hair fell out from the immunosuppressant aspect of the drug.

I had to mentally battle the pros and cons of this medication. I was experiencing more and more joint pain which didn't make a lot of sense to me. I was angry. I felt that life had robbed me, that my glorious years of youth were being stolen from me and I couldn't do anything about it.

I was then moved onto a combination of the DMARD and a biologic. This was when things started to look like they were going for the better. This new medication stopped the progression of my joint pain. While I still had a lot of pain, it stopped any new joints from flaring, and I was happy with that! I'm still on this combination drug, but it hasn't completely controlled my joint pain or my flares so, in the next few months I'll probably be moved onto a new medication.

During my sixth year in school – and of course with the leaving cert on the horizon – my RA reacted to this stressful environment. It seems anytime I have a test coming up or anything remotely important, my RA decides to have a temper tantrum and leaves me bed-ridden for days.

I've been battling this whole year with finding a happy medium between listening to my body and resting when I need rest and working through the pain, so as to not stress me out over the lack of work I was doing. I wish I could say I have found that happy medium, but not yet.

Right now, I'm in a state of mind where I evaluate each day as it comes and make accommodations accordingly and it seems to be working for me. I have learned and am still learning to register my pain and fatigue levels and not resent myself for however those levels may restrict me. I cannot change my condition; I cannot change that I may wake up and be in a huge amount of pain, but I can change how I react to it. I have learned to not panic; the work will eventually get done and one day in bed won't mean I will fail my exams. This is not my fault; this is just the situation I am in right now and I have to accept that.

Rheumatoid arthritis is an invisible illness. No one would ever look at me and think I have a chronic illness. This isn't always the most positive thing and I'm sure most people with RA can relate to this. Whenever I am talking to my friends about my condition, I always have this little voice in the back of my head calling me a liar and begging me to stop whinging.

It leads to this constant feeling that I have to validate my suffering and prove that I actually am in pain. I'm not in bed because I'm lazy and I'm not holding ice to my joints to get attention. This can all mean then that I have to cancel plans last minute or be careful about how often I go out. I then get told that I'm 'unreliable'. When really, I'm not unreliable, my illness is.

This can often be difficult to articulate to my friends and it isn't their fault that they don't understand. This is something that most 18 year olds don't understand and why should they?

That being said, I have gained so much from my experience with RA; I would not be the person that I am today without it and I am so grateful for that. I have learned that I'm resilient, that I have this reserve of power within me that I can tap into when I feel like I have nothing left. I have gained a strength that I never would have had if I didn't have RA.

My condition has also highlighted the amount of amazing, supportive people that I have in my life. I never would have made it through the tougher times without my family and friends. My mum has held me on the sofa more times than I can count and given me the reassurance and comfort that I needed. Every time that I have dug my heels in and given up on everything, she has picked me up and forced me to keep going. I will forever be in debt to her. I would never have gotten through the days when I was in school and in pain without my friends. The spontaneous hugs and encouraging words have been the driving force of getting me through all of this. I have an incredible support system around me and my RA has shown that to me and therefore, I am thankful for it.

I am still in the midst of a storm with my RA, I am in no way through it and in remission. However, I know I will get through it and I will make it to the other end. Besides, I kind of like that I have a bit of a story to tell!

Catherine O'Connor

When my work asked me to go to India for 10 days my heart sank, my son Sean was 10 months old and I didn't want to leave him, he was my world.

I protested but eventually relented and agreed to go, it was 2009, the recession was hitting and I was anxious to mind my job.

On the way home from work the day I was due to travel to India, somebody crashed into the back of me, Sean was in the car. The impact was serious enough, but no one was injured. I stuck to my plans to travel.

I set off on my flight to Bangalore, my mind raced, the stress of leaving Sean and the accident earlier that day had caught up with me. I wouldn't have thought it was humanly possible, but I cried all the way to Bangalore.

After the 13-hour flight, I literally couldn't move, it took all the strength I had to get off the plane. My joints had seized up. I got to the hotel and slept; when I woke up I wasn't much better. I got through the days in Bangalore thanks to kind colleagues and paracetamol. But for me the source of my aliments was not really a mystery, I recognised the symptoms, the movements, the agonising efforts to stand up, sit down, to clasp my hand around a cup of tea; I had grown up watching these movements. My mother had suffered from RA as well.

My worst nightmare was descending around me.

I cut my trip short and returned home after a week. I don't think I even remember the trip home, the pain and tiredness enveloped me. I went to see my GP, who agreed with my self-diagnosis, but took blood tests to confirm. He injected me with steroids. I went to bed in my own house that night, happy to be back with my precious boy – but terrified.

I had grown up with what was now my own future, I had seen the disease up close, I had hated this disease long before it had ravaged my own joints. I had known how my mother had suffered, I was sure this was my future. I was only 33 and I was imagining myself on a mobility scooter. It was hard to believe that two weeks before that I had thought I was a girl about town and now I was contemplating life as an invalid.

My whole life had changed. I had hope of having more children, my doctor advised me that this may not be as easy with my new diagnosis.

I found having RA was an exhausting disease. My consultant described it not a very sexy disease – he was right about that. This he explained was why there wasn't much time, money or effort spent on researching it in the '70s and '80s. This explains my mother's experience with the disease. He reassured me my outcome would be better. The new biologics were on the market in the last few years and he was hopeful that these would work for me. I heard the phrase 'fighting fire with fire' several times.

I limped, stiffly and sorely around, trying to pretend everything was normal. I didn't really talk about it, I thought I was hiding it. I was embarrassed to have arthritis. People looked at it as an old person disease, if I did mention it, people often told me that their grandmother, grandfather has arthritis in the knuckles, right hand, etc. They weren't trying to be unkind, but they didn't realise that the disease that was taking over my life was more than the aches and pains suffered by an octogenarian.

I preferred to keep the whole thing to myself. I had led a very healthy life up to this; the shock of not be able to do things for myself was very hard to deal with.

Thankfully, the new biologics did work. I eventually hit on the right one that suited me. I initially took it with a DMARD (disease-modifying anti-rheumatic drug), but after a few years came off this, due to some alarming liver functionality results.

But the biologics have been good to me. For 10 years I led a normal life only coming off them when trying to get pregnant, or when pregnant. The doctors were right, fertility and maintaining pregnancy was not so easy when suffering from a chronic disease.

But six years after my diagnosis, I had my beautiful Mathew and, a year after, my wonderful surprise baby Hannah. Due to some trickery of the body, arthritis totally disappears for many people throughout pregnancy and for some months after giving birth. I was one of these, so my two pregnancies were free from arthritis symptoms. And thankfully my nightmare of a mobility scooter has yet to be realised.

My mother's disease and symptoms have also eased up, due to the advances in medication in the last 10-20 years, yet she lives with deformities and disabilities that have been caused by the aggressive RA she has endured since her mid-40s. She is now nearly an octogenarian herself.

I count myself lucky that these medical advances are available now. I dread to think how my life would be if they weren't.

Amanda Prather

One summer morning in 2015, I awoke with an itch. It was in the centre of my back and as I attempted to perform the usual twists and turns to reach the elusive spot, I found myself greatly struggling. My body felt hardened, stiff well beyond anything I experienced before. Then I noticed my fingers were unusually inflexible, unable to bend with ease.

My mind scanned for any symptoms I could possibly attribute to this. The first to emerge: rheumatoid arthritis. I quickly disregarded this notion, unable to entertain even the idea of this possibility. It must be something else, a one-off occurrence. Ignoring my natural instincts, I moved forward, convinced the ailment that plagued my fears was ludicrous.

Nearly four years later, I find myself settling into life with rheumatoid arthritis. It's a new normal, the memories of my previous body daily drifting away.

My official diagnosis occurred in the spring of 2016. Though summer 2015 had been my first awareness of possible RA symptoms, I had already experienced a few unknowns earlier that spring – some fatigue, ankle swelling, minor pain in my knee joint.

Once autumn approached, things began deteriorating rapidly. I had just returned from a lengthy work trip to Africa and the travel and jet lag wrecked my body in ways that

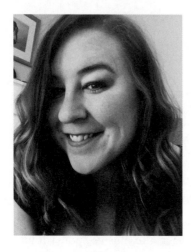

Amanda Prather

previous travelling had never done.

My ankles and feet felt like they were on fire, while simultaneously being gripped with the force of a giant as they throbbed in pain. During my worst moments, walking seemed like a luxury. Simple things like showering and using the toilet were tasks that required a period of mental preparation in order to endure the physical pain and exhaustion that came with it, often ending with me sobbing in frustration.

I'd never felt fatigue and pain like this before, both in description and intensity. There would be mornings when I would lie in bed, writhing in pain, and begging my body to heal. My mattress supporting my body, I lay there several times with such intense pain that I contemplated urinating in my own bed rather than endure the arduous task of using the toilet. To find myself in a situation where the pain was so strong that soiling myself was a better alternative than crawling 15 feet to the toilet was alarming.

In 2012, my mom lost her battle with leukaemia. Over the six years of her battle, I had formed an unhealthy fear of doctors and hospitals. Many of her visits left us holding our breath, preparing for the worst. When my own pain started, I found myself dismissing my concerns, my fear strengthened by my avoidance. Eventually I opened up to my sister and asked for her help.

I had been hiding it from everyone, partly from my fear to admit the depth of the problem, but also because I was too proud to admit I was hurting. When she realised how bad it had been, she began talking with me about going to the doctor, doing what she could to reassure me that we would deal with it together.

Summoning the courage to face a doctor took another month and when I did, my life was forever changed.

At 35, I learned that I had RA and in the past year, it had rapidly deteriorated my knee joint. Not only was I facing the diagnosis, but I had to have a total knee replacement. Less than a year prior, before the pain had started, I was running a couple of miles two or three times a week. Pain-free. Now my knee was done. I went to the doctor in mid-March and in the span of three weeks, I faced a new chronic illness and a major surgery.

The emotional toll it had on me was unexpected. After my mom lost her battle with cancer, I felt like nothing would phase me again. The thing I dreaded most in life happened and I survived. I lumped all of life's negative experiences together, believing I was now immune to them all. But I had lived dealing with my mom's illness, not my own. This presented an entirely different set of emotions – navigating through different types and levels of pain, loneliness and fear.

Processing through the emotions is a never-ending journey. I grieved deeply – for my old body, for my future and for who I would never be again. My carefree days were gone.

My choices now seemed controlled by my defunct

immune system. No more running. No more volleyball. Walks were a challenge. Energy was limited, not renewable. Fatigue became commonplace.

In the mirror, my body reflected a woman in her 30s, but inside I felt as if I had aged 40 years. The vibrancy and spontaneity I had felt in life was replaced by trepidation and anxiety. My focus was no longer on my experiences and the joy they brought to my life. Now it was filled with logistics: how far do I have to walk, will I have to stand for long, will there be physical exertion, is there seating for when I get tired, will I have time to rest, can I keep up? The things I had easily enjoyed in the past could now fill me with dread. My passion for travel, sports, concerts and fun activities waned – it felt as if a part of me was slowly dying.

Worry took hold, gripping and clawing its way into me, burrowing into my brain. My existence felt like a burden on the people in my life: present and future. I worried about how I held back my friends and family. Would they have more fun if I wasn't around? Did they wish I didn't come so they explore more? I wasn't married and wondered if I would find someone that would love me with a chronic illness. Would they regret being with someone that couldn't be as adventurous? What about the financial burden or the possible future of care taking? Could I enjoy the physical part of the relationship?

My brain swirled with unfounded and illogical worries. My friends and family were supportive, wonderful and loving. I was beyond blessed to have them in my life, yet my fears dominated. The challenge to quiet them down is ongoing, though it feels like I am moving into the winning side of this battle.

RA is an invisible illness. You can't see how it affects my

body or others', but it's there, lingering below the surface. Though it can occasionally feel like the exact opposite. If I limp because my ankle is flaring-up or when I have to sit at a party because I get too fatigued, I feel anything but invisible. It seems like a spotlight is on me with red lights flashing and a voice screaming 'She's not normal! She is different!' But most times, the invisible attribute is apt. You feel alone and that no one understands your situation. It's isolating and makes you retreat, allowing the invisibility to be your shield.

Thankfully, my journey has evolved over the years. Medicinal trial and errors left me drained and in much pain, fearful that nothing would ever work. Finally, my wonderful disease-modifying drug (DMARD) came into my life. I feel like I regained a lot of what I had lost. Not all of it – I will never be 100% again.

And though most of the barriers and limitations are still in place, it's lessened to a tolerable level. My fears still emerge as the concerns never fully diminish. Every new ache brings instant dread – belief that the disease is progressing.

But I am learning to navigate through it all. My confidence in my post-RA abilities and everyday achievements is growing. I am learning not to identify as a victim of a chronic illness, but as a person living with it. I won't allow my identity to become consumed by my immune system. I want to be challenged and strengthened by what I face in my life. Character is built through endurance and trials and I want my illness to become my greatest motivator rather than my biggest defeat.

Believing people with a chronic illness is important. When they are describing their pain, experiences and emotions, it's necessary to listen and trust their words.

Last year I moved from the US to Ireland for graduate school. I went to my last appointment with my US rheumatologist before moving and I struggled to hold back tears. My relationship with him was a normal and professional doctor-patient relationship. But my affection for him was lodged in his understanding and belief. He knew, within a touch of a joint, how badly I hurt. He knew my pain, he sympathised when I hurt, and he treated me.

Having someone that believes your pain, fatigue and struggles is invaluable. I realised he was the only person who truly understood what I faced. He made me feel less invisible. But hopefully, my story and others will change that.

Compassion abounds in this world. We just have to share who we are, what we are facing and how people can love and support this lifelong journey we are experiencing. My hope and belief is that people with RA won't be invisible much longer. We will be believed. We will be understood. And we will overcome.

Edwina Ryle

I'm writing this because when I was first diagnosed with rheumatoid arthritis, I had no idea what this meant or where to get help and support.

It would have been great to have read other stories to help me cope, to help me understand and to give me some idea of what to expect.

When my GP rang to say that my blood tests results were back and that I had RA, I was totally shocked. All I heard was the word 'arthritis' and to me arthritis was something only old people got! I was 47 at the time, with three young children. My GP told me there was a drug I could take and I would hardly know I had it. This isn't entirely true!

It took a few weeks to get an appointment with a consultant and it can be hard to find the right consultant. They need to be someone that you can relate to and that you like. This is someone that you will come to depend on and you will have many visits with before everything settles down. You need to be able to trust them and believe them. It's a big decision. It's hard to find out where to go and to get a good recommendation.

During this time, I was in a lot of pain, I was scared and there were so many unanswered questions. I had no idea what the future held for me. I suddenly felt very old. You take your

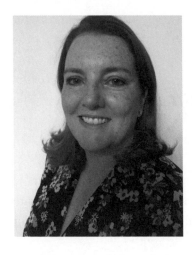

Edwina Ryle

health so much for granted until something goes wrong. The future didn't look so bright anymore. My diagnosis filled me with many emotions; fear, anger, guilt. Could I have done something to prevent this?

Once I met with my consultant, I felt more at ease. I was given a DMARD (disease-modifying anti-rheumatic drug) and steroids and was told that within 12 weeks I should feel a lot better.

Unfortunately, this relief was short lived. In my experience, GPs and consultants don't manage your expectations!

The pain didn't go away in 12 weeks, and for the next 14 months my dosage was repeatedly increased and new drugs were added. And while I felt better at times, I was far from perfect. Finding the right balance of drugs takes time. As well as the physical pain and discomfort, it is also emotionally draining.

There are many side effects to drugs, which you just have to put up with and over time you get used to them. Feeling nauseous, headaches and fatigue were the main side effects that I felt from all the drugs.

Another thing nobody tells you is how expensive this diagnosis is: consultant appointments, blood tests, x-rays, medication, physio, hydrotherapy – they add up.

At times, the pain was quite debilitating. I found myself struggling to do many everyday tasks such as driving, getting dressed, brushing my teeth, brushing/washing my hair and the list goes on.

It felt like every few days a different joint was affected. Just as one joint would be back to normal, another one would be affected. RA can be very random. My husband described it as dynamic!

I was also diagnosed with fibromyalgia around this time. RA and fibromyalgia often go hand in hand, so now I was dealing with a second problem. I often wonder would I have developed fibromyalgia in the first 12 months, if I hadn't been so stressed and so worried about my RA diagnosis.

The emotional pain was very draining too.

I felt guilty that I couldn't do everything as before. My energy levels were very low. I wasn't the wife or mother that I used to be, that I wanted to be. My children had to step up and help out a lot more in the house. I didn't want my children to be burdened with a mother who was unwell. My children were 13, 10 and 8 at the time.

In time, my children became more understanding and supportive, and we worked our way through it through humour. Although there are still days when I need to rest and my husband and children want me and expect me to be able to function normally!

My husband was always supportive, but he found it hard at times to know what to say to make me feel better. For a long time he was the only person I talked to about my diagnosis. It's not that it was a secret, but I was reluctant to give too many details. I played it down a lot. I felt nobody understood, as you always look perfectly normal and well. I didn't want sympathy. I didn't want to be judged. And most of all, I didn't want the free advice from people who hadn't a clue what they were talking about!

I also felt angry. Why me? What could I have done to prevent this? Is this genetic? Is it my age? Is it because I'm female? Will I ever get remission? So many unanswered questions.

I consoled myself by thinking it could be worse...

With RA you look absolutely fine, so people assume that therefore you must be fine.

Three years on, I feel a lot better. I am still on a lot of medication, including a biologic which is an injection I take weekly. The plan is now to reduce my medication over time, and I recently came off the steroids – that felt good!

The fatigue and other side effects have eased too.

I still have bad days, but they are less and less. I have struggled to meet people under the age of 50 with RA. Now I live my life as well as I can, taking the good days with the bad and try not to get too down when a bad day comes along.

The fact that this is a lifelong condition that isn't going to go away takes time to process and accept.

Allow yourself the time you need.

Don't put pressure on yourself and be resilient.

Gloria Shannon

The lump in my throat grew and I gave a half-smile, hoping that would satisfy their need to know I was ok. I prayed they would look away before the tears stung my eyes and escaped down my cheek. I stood at the edge of the lake watching them play and laugh. They hopped in and out of the little boat with ease. I tried to be happy for them, but instead I just felt sorry for myself.

You see, I was having a flare-up and even making it out as far as the lake was a big deal. However, in that moment I just wanted to be able to forget about RA. To jump, and laugh and play like the others. I was 26 years of age and I didn't have the energy or capability to get in and out of a boat.

So, yet again, I stood at the edge of that lake and grief waved over me again. Grief for the me that could have been. For what must be the one-hundredth time I grieved for the 26-year-old, the 15-year-old me dreamed about. And not for a second, did she ever consider the physical struggles the real 26-year-old would face. She dreamed of being a writer, a teacher, an interior designer, of travelling the world, partying all night with her friends and getting up the next day to do it all over again.

At 15, all those dreams changed, even if I didn't fully realise it then. First, there was a twinge in my knees. Next it

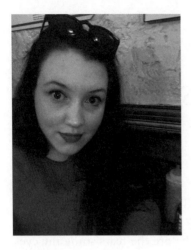

Gloria Shannon

was difficult to move my fingers, open doors, walking became difficult. I was terrified so I tried to bury my head in the sand and hoped that it would just go away. I had never experienced something like this before. Of course, my parents noticed a change in me and made me go to doctors. A lot of blood tests, x-rays, MRIs and hospital appointments later, I was told I had rheumatoid arthritis.

I didn't grieve then, because I don't think I understood the severity of it all. I was sure I was going to get medicine and in a few weeks, maybe months, I would be right as rain and back to normal. That is how doctors and medicines worked. They fixed you.

That wasn't the case. 'Manage' and 'lifelong illness' were the words thrown around. I remember hearing them and I also remember discarding them to the back of my mind.

My life had changed, but I lived in hope that medicine would cure all. It definitely helped at first. Still my day to day life was very different. It wasn't until my leaving cert year, I began to grieve for the future me I had lost.

Sitting on my bed with my arms raised as my sister put

my t-shirt on me like she was dressing a baby. A big, adult-sized baby. In that moment, I think I grieved for the first time. It just hit me that I was never going to have the life I had imagined and I was never going to be that carefree teenager that took her health for granted again.

I didn't understand that it was grief at the time. I thought grief was something you experienced solely after losing a loved one. I never realised you could grieve for other things in life, your marriage, your job… your health.

Due to my health, I watched all my friends go to college and I was left behind. I had dreamed of college for as long as I could remember and, yet again, my health was holding me back. I just wasn't in a place to go full-time. That stung.

College was all I ever wanted. I don't think I had really even thought past that point. I just knew I loved learning and there I would be given a wealth of knowledge and inspiration. Instead, I was at home, trying to become well enough to go to further education full-time.

Since then, I have grieved many times for the me that was and the me that was going to be. I won't ever climb Everest, I won't ever be the strongest person in the room and my life is harder that most at 27 years of age. And like grief for a loved one, I have come to the point of acceptance.

I have accepted that this is my life, I go further to say I think I have embraced it. I write about my experiences of living with this illness, both the sad and funny (yes, there can be humour in it all). I volunteer with arthritis groups and try to help others come to terms with their illness in any way I can.

I also got well enough to go to college and get my degree; one of the proudest moments of my life. Being able to achieve that showed me how much is still possible with this illness.

So most days, I don't grieve, not after 12 years of having RA, I just get on with it. It's my new normal. To be honest, it has been this long that I don't really remember much of a way of life without it. It is just a part of me. And in honesty how I deal with it, how I have dealt with it taught me so much about empathy and respect and humour. I truly believe it has ultimately made me a better person having to go through my teens and 20s with this hurdle to overcome time and time again.

Still, there are times I sit on my bed trying to get dressed, slowly, in pain... or a moment where I am standing on the sidelines, watching my friends play fight, or that day when I have to call in sick... that the grief hits me.

It knocks me for six, right in the chest, and I can feel the tears about to sting my eyes and the lump in my throat. In that moment I am taken back to sitting on the bed at the age of 18 while my younger sister dressed me. It might be a few minutes or hours, but it feels like I have to go through the whole process again.

Time heals all wounds.

Whilst no amount of time will heal me, cure me, fix me... it does help. Time makes it easier to cope with. Time may not have completely healed my wound, but it has eased the pain. Hopefully it will continue to as I grow older and wiser I become more and more confident that, sure, I have arthritis...

But arthritis doesn't have me.

Paul H. Tubb

I am a humourist. I write rhymes, occasional prose, songs and draw pictures with the hopes that once heard/seen by someone, they will provoke laughter within that person. I have performed my work to many children around the island of Ireland and received a pleasant response. I like to think of myself as a funny person.

When someone is known for being funny, it is often said of them, that they have 'funny bones'. Well as a sufferer of rheumatoid arthritis, I'm often reminded just how unfunny and humourless my bones can be.

My first experience with RA, was not my own. My maternal grandmother suffered herself from this affliction, and I was to receive a memory that has stuck with me all my life. My grandmother died in 1979 when I was 6 years old, so obviously this memory is from a long time ago, when I was very young.

A person's memory being what it is, an unreliable record keeper that can make changes/additions at will, this tale may have the occasional over-embellishment or even under-embellishment; it could be more traumatic than I remember or less, but the following is how I remember it.

My granny and I were sitting in a small space with a stage. I will not be so grandiose as to call it a theatre, because

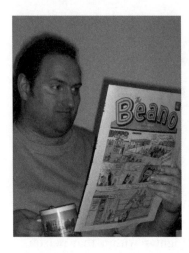

Paul H. Tubb

I believe it was a church hall transformed into a theatre, for the performance that afternoon. My elder sister and brother were performing as part of an Irish dancing competition.

Being a pastime I did not indulge in, I was out in the audience. I can only assume that my mother was backstage, preparing my older siblings for the event and calming the nerves for the obvious crowd roar and adulation forthcoming.

I was the youngest, my now younger brother having not yet been born. I have very fond memories of my granny and she was very fond of me; so being left alone with her was normally a most pleasant experience, one we both enjoyed.

Yet this instance was not the pleasant occurrence I had been exposed to up to now. Her hand was set in a claw-like grasp. She told me she was unable to move her fingers straight. I thought she was teasing me, and I said, 'Yes you can.'

She then offered me the opportunity to try and see if I was able to move them. I, of course, could not. I knew automatically that this was not right. She wasn't deliberately preventing me from moving them, she genuinely couldn't move her fingers. This traumatised and scared me. My granny had exposed a frailty that I had difficulty comprehending. Why couldn't she move her fingers?

My young mind tried to comprehend. This was not right, there must be something wrong with her. I dealt with this, the way you would expect someone with my lack of years and maturity would.

I screamed, yelled, cried and caused a tremendously unholy scene that was probably only assuaged by the offer of sweets or a comic.

Years later I discovered she suffered from rheumatoid arthritis, but not realising this was a genetic condition, I didn't worry too much about that news.

Fast forward to around 2014/2015. I, having moved to Ireland from my native UK in 2002, was living in Howth, Co. Dublin and working in Dublin's city centre. I started to experience numb pains in my hands, wrist, back and thighs. At first I thought very little of this, 'it'll pass' was my general thought. Even though it was making drawing (my favourite pastime) and playing the guitar uncomfortable, I was still hoping for a natural end.

The pain did not subside. It started to get so bad that the pain would wake me up at ridiculously early times in the morning, necessitating the need to get out of bed; as lying there was contributing to my discomfort.

I would take a painkiller, usually to no avail. Then I would make myself a cup of coffee, prepare a hot water bottle, put a DVD on (I was going through a *Classic Doctor* phase at the time) and then lie on the sofa with the hot water bottle on the part of my anatomy that was giving me the most distress, before moving it to the next anatomical part. Eventually I had to make my way to work, although I did miss the odd day.

My stubbornness had to give way. I was losing sleep and

making my wife's life harder and she had her own health issues. I finally went to my GP, and he told me it could be RA. It was a genetic disease, he said, and asked about my family history. I informed him about my grandmother, although left out the traumatic way I found out. He wrote a letter and told me to go straight to Beaumont Hospital.

I was registered, my bloods were taken and then I was told to go to the rheumatology department at a certain time. When I was seen, the doctor inspected my knuckles and hands and she told me that she didn't believe it was RA, as my hands were not showing the inflammatory signs usually associated with the disease.

She called a colleague and he said the same. They told me that my blood work would give more of a picture as to what my ailment was, but they were adamant that none of the outward physical signs of RA were apparent, so it probably wasn't that.

I was both relieved and worried. I was relieved that I probably didn't have rheumatoid arthritis, and would never have to put up with what my poor grandmother had to deal with. But was worried as I had no idea what it could be.

Eventually I was told that it was, in fact, rheumatoid arthritis; but it was in such an early stage that my outward appearance was showing no signs of it.

This surprised me as I had waited a long time before I saw the doctor regarding my pains, but this lack of advancement pleased me. Something that pleased me more, was being told that since 1979, the advances in medical science means that I could now take daily medicine that would treat my symptoms and alleviate my suffering.

Recently I learned from my physician that medical science advancements were not without their pitfalls.

It was revealed to me that the DMARD (disease-modifying anti-rheumatic drug) I was prescribed for the treatment of my RA, negatively affects eyesight and can cause blindness in certain cases. I discovered this after taking it for some time, and having it alleviate a lot of my RA symptoms satisfactorily. So I'm still taking that drug, but also taking care of my eyes as well, with yearly visits to the opticians.

And that is where I am today, taking pills and making regular trips to the hospital to see if my bloods tell a different story.

Life is more tolerable now, but every so often, my bones can't help themselves reminding me how unfunny and humourless they are. These occasions are rarer now, but I have discovered an ice pack works a lot better than a hot water bottle.

One thing I'd like to say to anyone reading this, is if you feel numb pains in your joints or thigh, go straight to a doctor. If you have RA, it can be treated and if you catch it early, it will be the better for it. Also, take care of your eyes.

Mary Whelan

Where do I begin, or indeed how do I begin to tell you a story of how rheumatoid arthritis changed my life?

I was diagnosed at the age of 37. I woke up one morning with stiffness in my fingers, they were very hard to move or to make a fist. This was one of many symptoms I had before I was diagnosed.

Many a time as I walked up my hometown of Arklow, I would have to stop as my ankle gave me so much pain. This happened at random times. I used to think that people might think I was a bit mad as I limped for a while, then it would be gone. I found this very frustrating.

Prior to these aches and pains, I was a marathon runner and was extremely fit. I used walk a mile to my aerobics class, do a strenuous work out, run maybe three miles and walk another mile back home. Or I might often run 10k without a thought.

When I developed this debilitating disease, everything changed. I was so down in myself; I became dependant on my family, couldn't open a jar, tie my shoes, fasten my bra or wash my hair.

I found myself in so much pain, from the tip of my head to my toes. Pain 24/7 caused me to feel hopeless. I was, and indeed am, very lucky to have my husband John and

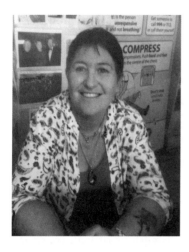

Mary Whelan

my children William, Róisín and Niamh to care for me, if I needed it.

Once I was diagnosed, the consultant in St Vincent's put me on a DMARD (disease-modifying anti-rheumatic drug), but after three months, I was getting worse.

At this stage, I couldn't walk, my feet were so swollen my shoes didn't fit. I could not lift my arms or bend my wrists without severe pain.

It was obvious to my consultant that this medication was failing me.

It was then that I was asked to spend some time in Our Lady's Hospice, Harold's Cross, which has a dedicated rheumatology unit. I spent two weeks there, getting daily physio and hydro pool exercises. It was a great benefit.

I also learned about and was put on a biologic drug, which has helped me so much, that most of my pain vanished. I was back to myself. My life was wonderful again, I wasn't running marathons, but I could walk without pain.

After 12 years on this treatment, then to my horror, my body became immune to it. After several failed experiments, I found a different treatment that is working for me now.

Many of my joints are damaged and some day, I will need surgery. I'm well aware of this.

There are other challenges; I also have osteoarthritis, bursitis, fibromyalgia and inflammation in the sternum. I have blood tests every three months to monitor my liver and kidneys in case of any side effects from the medication. I find that I'm very tired at times and don't want to do much sometimes.

Along with the physical side effects, there is also the mental health side. People look at me and tell me I look great, but every morning it's difficult to get out of bed; there are times I just don't want to.

So, I push myself a lot. Maybe too much, then I suffer the next day, but if I don't use my joints, I will 'lose' them.

To finish my story, I'm 55 now and while some of my joints are damaged, I'm still here, alive and at least look well. I'm an artist and love to write poetry, so I keep myself busy.

It is important to get an early assessment, to look after yourself and respect your joints. Most of all, do as your consultant suggests and the light at the end of the tunnel will become brighter.

Arthritis Ireland

Arthritis Ireland is the national patient organisation representing one million people – including 1,200 children and young people – living with arthritis in this country.

Our vision is of a better life for people living with arthritis today and a world without arthritis tomorrow.

Arthritis Ireland is working in communities across the country providing education and support to help people effectively manage their condition, to remove the pain and social isolation caused by the disease and to ensure people remain active and doing the things they love. We undertake grassroots advocacy and public engagement, so that the voice of people with arthritis is heard and understood, as well as investing in research to find better treatments and ultimately a cure.

To find out how Arthritis Ireland can support you or someone you love, **visit www.arthritisireland.ie, call our helpline on 01 661 8188 or 1890 252 846** or **email helpline@arthritisireland.ie**.